# SHIFT
# STRESS

*Get Back to What you do Best:
for Nurses, Caregivers and other
Health Care Professionals*

*By Vij Richards*

To Craig & Aline
with thanks for the
great work & Contribution
you offer us all!  Vij ♡

◆ FriesenPress

Suite 300 - 990 Fort St
Victoria, BC, V8V 3K2
Canada

www.friesenpress.com

ISBN
978-1-5255-5225-0 (Hardcover)
978-1-5255-5226-7 (Paperback)
978-1-5255-5227-4 (eBook)

*Self-Help, Self-Management, Stress Management*

Disclaimer:
The author of this book does not dispense medical advice or prescribe the use of any
technique as a form of treatment for physical, emotional, or medical problems
without the advice of a physician, either directly or indirectly. The intent of the
author is only to offer information of a general nature to help you in your quest
for emotional well-being. In the event that you use any of the information in
this book for yourself or others, the author assumes no responsibility for your
actions. All stories in this book are true. The names and circumstances of the
stories have been changed to protect the anonymity of all clients.

Cover Design: Friesen Press
Editing: Carolyn Wilker/Friesen Press
Author's photo courtesy of Rhona Haas Photography

Distributed to the trade by The Ingram Book Company

# TABLE OF CONTENTS

# ADVANCE PRAISE

We are thrilled to see Vij Richards bringing energy medicine and other integrative methods to nurses and other front line caregivers. Stress has been called "Public Health Enemy #1," and Shift Stress offers you powerful tools for understanding and countering the stresses you face within yourself and in your patients.

Donna Eden and David Feinstein
Co-authors, *The Energies of Love*

"This book offers insight in to attachment styles as a way to improve relationships under stress in the workplace."

Diane Poole Heller Ph.D., L P C, SEP, developer of the DAre method (dynamic attachment repatterning experience)
Diane Poole-Heller Ph.D

In Shift Stress, Vij Richards offers health care professionals a vital resource to minimize the impact of workplace stress and trauma. Her well-researched information and powerful suite of simple techniques provide these essential workers with hope and power to avoid and recover from the devastating impact of the compassion fatigue prevalent in these fields.

Ms. Richards engages the reader by sharing her personal story of burn out and recovery and then compassionately invites them to address their own stress issues using her proven strategies. Nurses and all health care professionals will find understanding and compassion and real help in Shift Stress.

I am honoured to be included as one of Ms. Richards' teachers of Emotional Freedom Techniques (EFT) and I am delighted that she has highlighted the power of EFT to support the quality of life of health care professionals.

Nancy Forrester
MBA, B.ED., B.Sc.
Clinical Member Ontario Society of
Psychotherapists (retired)
Accredited Master EFT Trainer of
Trainers (EFTInternational)
Executive Director, National Emotional Freedom
Techniques Training Institute

In Shift Stress Vij Richards offers concrete tools for recognizing and coping with the stressors of working in healthcare today. With stories and research-based evidence, she provided solutions that include abundant resources, actionable strategies, and alternative therapies to improve ourselves and our workplaces. This book will help and heal nurses and all healthcare workers.

LeAnn Thieman
Author of Chicken Soup for the
Nurse's Soul and SelfCare for HealthCare®

*In memory of my Mum and for all nurses and caregivers to support finding strength within themselves*

# A NOTE ABOUT
## Dragonflies

I've always loved dragonflies for their delicate, translucent wings and colourful bodies. I have a decorative dragonfly hanging off the bricks outside our home. I have two pillows with dragonflies on them that sit on the bench inside our red front door. I even own a tee shirt with a dragonfly on it. So, I was very excited to find out the spiritual meaning of dragonflies.

**Did you know that in almost every part of the world, the dragonfly symbolizes change, transformation, adaptability and self-realization?**

The change that is referred to often has its source in mental and emotional maturity, and in understanding the deeper meaning of life. The dragonfly's scurrying flight across water represents an act of going beyond what's on the surface and looking into the deeper implications and aspects of life. The dragonfly moves with elegance and grace. The dragonfly is iridescent, both on its wings and on its body. Iridescence shows itself in different colours, depending on the angle, and how the light hits it. The magical property of iridescence is also associated with the discovery of one's abilities by unmasking the real self and removing the doubts one casts on his/her own sense of identity.

The dragonfly lives most of its life as a nymph for up two years. It flies only for a fraction of its life, up to six months. This symbolizes and exemplifies the virtue of living in the moment and living life to the fullest. By living in the moment, you are aware of who you are, where you are, what you are doing, what you want, and what you don't want, and you make informed choices on a moment-to-moment basis. The eyes of the dragonfly symbolize the uninhibited vision of the mind and the ability to see beyond the limitations of the human self. Dragonflies can be a symbol of the self that comes with maturity. They can symbolize going beyond self-created illusions that limit our growth and our ability to change.

**The dragonfly has been a symbol of happiness, new beginnings and changes for many centuries. The dragonfly means hope, change and love.**

(https://dragonflytransitions.com/why-the-dragonfly/ 2019)

# A NOTE ABOUT THE BOOK

I was drawn to start writing a book in 2017. At that time, I had been working for over a decade in an acute care hospital setting. I had started my nursing career in a small community hospital in ICU/CCU and then on to Long Term Care. Both experiences left me with a desire to find a way to help people before they became sick or injured. That's when I discovered the speciality in nursing called Occupational Health. I loved the focus on prevention and health teaching. So, I left the hospital environment to become a certified occupational health nurse and practiced for the next decade in different industrial settings before I got an opportunity to return to a large community hospital.

My role as a clinic nurse in occupational health was, among other things, to assess injuries and illness of the staff in the hospital and to make a care plan to support them. I was not prepared for the emotional traumas and the conflicts at work and at home that people needed help with. I began to feel the need to find a way to help the staff experiencing these stressors in the workplace–something I was not familiar with in my own experience on the front line and something I didn't receive training in as a nurse. For example, how do you support yourself while working in a stressful, fast paced and often traumatic environment? In my search for quick and easy-to-learn tools, I came across Emotional Freedom Techniques—EFT.

I was so inspired by the changes that EFT produced in my own life that I wanted to share this technique with others.

At the time, it was an experiential therapy and a new way of releasing stress and feeling it shift in your body. It was quite subjective with little science to support it nor any studies to document the benefits of this tapping technique. Because EFT was not yet evolved enough to get the attention of mainstream medicine, I knew that it would not be acceptable to offer it in the workplace. Behind the scenes I did offer it, however, and it worked for others, too. In the meantime, I returned to school to get the credentials I needed to support my desire to either increase the hours I was counselling with the staff or start my own practice.

I became a Registered Psychotherapist, graduating in 2012 from Transformational Arts College in Toronto, the same year that EFT became an evidence-based tool. I gradually took off my nursing hat but was able to stay in occupational health to provide counselling to the staff of the hospital. I love helping people feel better about themselves and empowering them to make choices in difficult situations– choices that feel good for them.

After a while, I saw the same concerns repeated over and over– conflict with a co-worker or spouse, not feeling valued by a manager, grief of a family loss or patient tragedy. They all had one thing in common. What people were experiencing was emotional dysregulation (i.e. imbalance) and they were having difficulty tolerating this. They wanted to get back to feeling regulated (i.e. balanced) again and return to doing what they did best, in their jobs and their lives.

I began to have a desire to help more people and wondered if I could put what I had learned from my studies into a book. If so, I thought that I might be able to reach more health care professionals looking for help to support themselves and that they wouldn't take as long to find relief as I did. So, I began writing this book and what I thought would be helpful for others ended up giving me more clarity on my own journey. I'm always amazed how the universe creates these synchronistic opportunities that surround us when we are open to stepping out of our comfort zone to try something new and the road opens to guide us where to go next.

In this book, I have chosen to use a main character I have called "Kim" to represent many of my client's stories and to protect their identity. Kim has a problem to solve. She's struggling with workplace stress and relationship stress at work and at home—a situation that affects many nurses, probably all over the world. Kim needs help learning strategies to cope and strategies to work through solutions to her problems. Wouldn't it be nice to have a tool box of coping strategies to use when in need?

I, too, have struggled with stressful situations at work and home. I have included some of my own story of finding my voice and the tools that helped me to get to where I am today in order to illustrate some learning points in the chapters. Perhaps you are ready to update your own tool box? If so, this book is for you.

Kim is represented as a female character, but many of the examples could easily be male. There is a welcome increase of males entering the nursing profession and this book is for them, too. Where I have named a nurse in a story, it could as easily be any health care provider, such as personal support workers, pharmacists, porters, lab techs, physicians, physiotherapists, occupational therapists or dietary staff. In fact, any person in a role that involves patient care has the potential to be affected by the patient/caregiver relationship.

Each chapter features a different theme about stress and includes information to support that focus. The information given may provide insight into your own situation and how that increased awareness might help you manage your next stressful moment. At the end of each chapter, you'll find exercises that will help you to shift that stress.

In the context of this book, "shift stress" means going from a disempowered state to an empowered one– to regaining a sense of control. It helps you to get unstuck by shifting whatever is showing up as a challenge to you and changing a thought or behaviour to clear that challenge so that you can hear, see or feel it differently. When your inside world changes, the way you see things on the outside also changes.

**Caring for others is such a satisfying job and it shouldn't come at the expense of our own health.**

Let's be role models for all health care providers by making a difference in the way we care for ourselves and each other.

The World Health Organization (WHO) has designated 2020 as the year of the Nurse and Midwife in honour of the 200th anniversary of Florence Nightingale's birthday on May 12, 1820.

And coincidentally and timely the theme for National Nursing week 2020 is, "A Voice to Lead – Nursing the World to Health" So, with your empathy to connect with another person and your compassion to care, let your voice empower you to make a difference.

As well, on March 11, 2020, the WHO classified COVID-19 as a pandemic and the outbreak is evolving as I have come to the completion of my book. I would really like to hear from anybody reading this book to know if some of the techniques provided were of help to get you through some of your difficult days and to read about what has inspired you in this time of unprecedented social stress and global health crisis.

You can send your stories to: ShiftStress@gmail.com

# CHAPTER 1:
# What does a healthy work environment mean to you?

*"A healthy work environment is [...]*
*a practice setting that maximizes the health*
*and well-being of nurses, quality patient/client*
*outcomes, organizational performance, and*
*societal outcomes."*

—*Registered Nurses' Association of*
*Ontario (RNAO) March 2010*

Kim is eight hours into a twelve-hour shift when she starts to feel light-headed. She suddenly realizes that she hasn't yet been to the bathroom and she hasn't eaten anything. Then, coming around the corner, she hears her clinical department educator gathering staff for an in-service on ways to cope with stress.

It used to be that, once in a while, Kim had a crazy shift but now it seems every day is like this—it's becoming the norm.

Kim is worn down. She goes to the bathroom, gets her lunch and dutifully attends the in-service. In the back of her mind, she's thinking of her patient who has been vomiting all day and will likely be in a state by the time this session is over. And then there's the guy who has been calling for his meds and they're not due for another hour. There are so many people needing her attention. So much to do and not enough time, and now Joyce, her clinical educator, has invited some lady to talk to the team about stress!

Kim goes home that night, late, after reporting about her patient's day to the oncoming nurse and getting her charting caught up. She starts to reflect on her day. She's giving everything she's got and it just doesn't seem to be enough. Giving a hundred and ten percent to patients seems to be taking ten percent off her life. She doesn't feel alone; she knows her friends at work feel the same way. She's been on the same unit for ten years now and has shared stories with her co-workers as their families have grown up together. They used to go watch games together and socialize but that doesn't happen much anymore. She feels sad about that.

She checks on her kids. One is snuggled on the couch watching TV with her dad and the other is on the phone with her boyfriend. Kim smiles, grateful to come home to a loving husband and healthy kids. Her husband looks up and smiles, "I've got this stain on my shirt that I can't get out. Do you mind taking a look at it for me? Oh! And your sister called. She didn't sound good. She asked if you'd give her a call when you got home."

She's just walked in the door, exhausted, and there is more giving to do before her day is done. Kim has a restless night and the words from the in-service she attended earlier that day run through her mind. "Breathe to relax and calm your mind," "Talk it out," "Ask for help," and "Be mindful and compassionate to yourself." She drifts off to sleep thinking: *I've got six hours and it starts all over again.*

How long can she keep this up? She has seen some of her co-workers going off work sick on a "stress leave" and she doesn't want to join them.

\* \* \*

**According to the Canadian Nurses Association (CNA), health is said to be a human right, accessible to all. In March 2006, the CNA defined health as "a state of complete physical, mental, social and spiritual well-being, and not merely the absence of disease or infirmity."**

The Ontario Hospital Association (2007) stated that health is much more than the absence of illness; it is an important force in our daily lives. It is influenced by life circumstances, beliefs, actions, culture and social, economic and physical environments.

Health is a vehicle that enables and facilitates meaningful living. Statistics Canada conducted the National Survey of the Work and Health of Nurses survey in 2005, in partnership with the Canadian Institute for Health Information and Health Canada (CIHI). This was the first survey of its kind to focus on the working conditions and health of Canadian nurses.

Statistics Canada surveyed a total of 18,676 nurses, including Licensed Practical Nurses (LPN), Registered Nurses (RN), and Registered Practical Nurses (RPN) in a variety of health care settings in all provinces and territories.

Highlights taken from that survey include that the average nurse in 2005 was 44.3 years old. The report also shares that substantial numbers of nurses worked overtime, with an average of four unpaid overtime hours each week. Only fifty-two percent of nurses thought there was enough staff to get the work done and provide quality patient care, leaving forty-eight percent who didn't share that belief.

Nearly half (forty-eight percent) of nurses who provided direct care reported having experienced a needlestick or other sharps injury from an object that had been contaminated by use on an infected patient.

Three in ten nurses reported that a patient had physically assaulted them in the previous year.

Emotional abuse from patients was even more commonly reported at forty-four percent.

Forty-four percent of female nurses and fifty percent of male nurses confided that they were exposed to hostility from co-workers. This is high, compared to the general population—among which just under thirty percent of people surveyed reported being exposed to hostility or conflict from co-workers.

Interestingly, the overwhelming majority of nurses (eighty-eight percent) were satisfied with their jobs.

Under risk factors, the report showed that in the previous twelve months, thirty-seven percent of nurses had experienced pain—while doing their regular work-related tasks of bending, pushing, pulling and lifting—serious enough to prevent them from carrying out their normal daily activities.

Depression was more common in nurses than in the general population of employed people and, as a consequence, medication use was more common among nurses.

Sixty percent of nurses had been away from work for health-related reasons in the year prior to the survey. Those who had been off missed an average of nearly twenty-four days over the year.

Stats Canada website posted that the total days lost per worker in a year in the public sector for both sexes in 2019 was fourteen point nine days and the private sector was nine days.

It was noted that nurses who worked the evening shift had a higher likelihood of experiencing fair or poor general health compared to nurses who usually worked the day shift.

Numerous interpersonal or psychological elements of the job were also related to fair or poor mental health or general health. These included high job strain (meaning the demands on the employee are high, but freedom to make decisions and use skills is low), low supervisor support, low co-worker support, low autonomy, poor nurse-physician working relations, lack of respect from superiors and high turnover of roles affecting team effectiveness.

The demands on the nurse, who is at the hub of all patient activity, is ever increasing, with demands coming from management, peers and co-workers, patients, patients' families and visitors.

## Where do we go from here?

We are facing a dilemma in healthcare. Maybe it's always been this way and I'm just recognizing this in my later years, but healthcare delivery certainly seems to be becoming more challenging. Each decade brings new ideas about what health is, and how to obtain it. Information and technology, the extensive array of medical tests, people's expectation that they will live longer and receive full work-ups and treatments to maintain their health– these all add a cost and burden to our communities. The complex choices in care also create more ethical questions that challenge our health care providers. Who gets to have the latest test? At what age? And what gender? There is unequal access to services depending on where we live. Of course, all families want what's best for their loved ones and it's very distressing to see anyone suffer. The health care system is being reformed to address many of these concerns and while that is going on, the day-to-day business of care is expected to continue, at a standard that people have come to expect.

When we step back and look at the bigger picture of how stress affects nurses and health care workers, we realize that it can affect not just their lives and the lives of their family members, but also the organizations they work for and, ultimately, patient care.

There has been no follow up to the National Study of 2005 but there continues to be concerns about the working conditions of health care workers and numerous studies on bullying, harassment and workplace violence that provides evidence that working conditions remains an ongoing issue.

The Canadian Federation Nurses Union (CFNU) has partnered with the University of Toronto's School of Nursing on the first anonymous nationwide assessment of the realities of nurses' work environments in every health sector, whether in hospitals, home care, the community or long-term care. Their aim is to present a snapshot of what is happening in hospital wards, in the community and in long-term care facilities on a daily basis in the wake of hearing from members about a deepening crisis of care. The survey was completed in 2019 and results are pending.[1]

---

1    https://nursesunions.ca/

It will be interesting to see if and how the profession has changed and what the future recommendations will be to support the challenges we are all facing, whether providing care or needing care.

Although our work within the system is ever-changing and health care delivery has many partners, there is a responsibility for governance and senior leadership within our organizations for how operations within the system will provide support for all its health care providers. The fast pace of the hospital environment creates gaps in communication between workers, departments, programs and partnerships.

This situation reminds me of the principles we were taught in occupational health nursing when looking at control strategies designed to minimize harm to workers from hazardous substances. Where possible, the hazard should be eliminated and, if this is not possible, then the hazard is replaced or substituted, along with implementing ways to increase safety; this includes everything from equipment to education. The last resort is to look for personal protection for the worker to keep them safe and well at work.

In this hierarchical order, the system changes to support the worker. What if the system, under constant pressure, is not able to support all of its workers? What if some workers fall into the gaps or get left behind?

My goal for this book is to look at us, as individuals, supporting our health care delivery system through its challenges and changes and to suggest that we can shift inside ourselves to bring hope and resilience and support to each other in our ongoing efforts to care for others.

# CHAPTER 2:
# Face your stress and take the test

*"without mental health there can be no true physical health"*

—*Bulletin of the World Health Organization 2013*

We live in an information age, where technology is exploding in our work, in our homes, and taking over how we relate to each other. It is imperative that we find a way to press the pause button at some point in every day. We recognize that stress is part of our daily life, good and bad, and when the daily stressors are not addressed, and are instead avoided, the accumulation can damage our health and the lives we lead.

If we don't stop to recognize the signs and learn to support each other under stress, we add greater strains and unrealistic expectations as we perform our roles, both at work and away from it. Stress can lead to more good people getting sick and burned out. As the statistics show, something needs to change.

The Centre for Addiction and Mental Health (in Toronto) states that, in any given week, half a million Canadians are unable to work because of mental illness and 355,000 are off-work on disability. The Mental Health Commission of Canada reports that one in five individuals will have a mental illness this year and, of these, only one in three will ask for help because of the stigma that still exists.

As a young mom working full time, I was one of these silent sufferers who did not ask for help. I was afraid to admit there was something wrong with me. I rationalized the situation and felt I could do better if I just tried harder. To me, everybody else looked like they were coping okay. *It must have been me. Maybe I wasn't good enough.*

So, the negative thoughts kept going around and around in my head. That was over thirty years ago and it's sad to see that mental stigma remains an issue today.

If we, as health care providers are having difficulty dealing with and talking about mental health, how can we expect to help our greater community to have that open conversation? The National Survey of the Work and Health of Nurses (2005) found that an aging workforce, working overtime, shortage of staff, injuries, physical and emotional abuse, pain, anxiety and depression were all issues at that time, and from my observations, these continue to challenge health care delivery today. There is hope for a more open conversation with millennials in our workplace—those people between ages eighteen to thirty-five—who will constitute half the global workforce by 2020.[2] The survey goes on to say that millennials who experience the same stressors resulting in mental health issues will be more likely to talk openly to advocate for change that supports mental health in the workplace.

## Stress in the helping professions

In 2013, the Mental Health Commission of Canada launched the National Standard of Canada for Psychological Health and Safety in the Workplace. This voluntary standard encourages workplaces to implement and continually improve support for a safe environment for workers' mental health.

Hans Selye, MD, PhD (1907-1982), the "Father of Stress," was a Hungarian endocrinologist and the first to give a scientific explanation for biological "stress." He borrowed the term "stress" from physics to describe an organism's physiological response to perceived stressful events in the environment.

The term "stress," as it is currently used, was coined by Hans Selye in 1936, who defined it as "the non-specific response of the body to any demand for change."[3]

---

2    2015 Sun Life Canadian Health Index

3    https://www.stress.org/what-is-stress

Acknowledging that stress is an inevitable part of our lives and our work, we need to learn to self-reflect regularly to observe how we are being affected by the work we do. It makes sense to start by facing our stress.

I recommend using the professional quality of life indicator, ProQOL, which is a free screening tool that helps individuals understand the type of stress they may be experiencing from a work perspective, whether compassion fatigue, vicarious trauma or burnout. The test is available at ProQOL.org.[4]

From the ProQOL screening tool, compassion satisfaction describes the pleasure we derive from being able to do our work well. It can be a feeling of positivity about our ability to contribute to our colleagues, to our work and to the wellbeing of our communities.

The research on "compassion fatigue" began in 1995 with Charles Figley, PhD, and has since included the similar terms "caregiver fatigue" and "empathy fatigue," for example. To date, there is no agreed upon universal term that fully encompasses these similar ideas.

Caregiver fatigue or *"Compassion fatigue (CF) refers to the profound emotional and physical exhaustion that helping professions and caregivers can develop over the course of their careers as helpers. It is a gradual erosion of all the things that keep us connected to others in our caregiver role: our empathy, our hope, and of course our compassion—not only*

---

4    The ProQOL tool by Beth Hudnall Stamm, PhD 2009

*for others, but also for ourselves."*[5] The inability to refuel can often result in physical and emotional exhaustion, frustration, anger and often depression.

This described me in the 1980s. Giving to my family and work, while going back to school was all do-able, or so I thought. I was running on four to five hours of sleep a night, I ate when I could stop for a bite, and my meals were often unbalanced. I had no exercise routine; I smoked a pack of cigarettes a day and I had no time for a social life. One day, my life came crashing to a halt when I had fallen asleep out of exhaustion from a twelve-hour night shift and my kids were playing outside, unsupervised. My adventurous six-year-old daughter decided to climb the apple tree in our yard. She took a tumble and I heard her anxiously calling out for me. She needed my help and I was slow to respond. My neighbour gladly came over to take care of the other three little ones while I made myself get out of bed to take my daughter to the hospital. Hours later, X-rays confirmed that my daughter had a fractured arm. For me, this was a wake-up call—I needed some time off to re-evaluate the life I was leading.

*"Vicarious traumatization (VT) is a term that was coined by Laurie Anne Pearlman and Karen Saakvitne to describe the profound shift that workers experience in their world view*

---

5    Mathieu, Françoise. The Compassion Fatigue Workbook. Routledge Taylor & Francis Group 2012, pg 8

*when they work with clients who have experienced trauma.*"[6] I had a client I'll call Martha. She was an ER nurse. Her manager called me, concerned that she was being short with co-workers and not performing as her usual self. She was very capable and strong, and she came to see me unwillingly. Fortunately, she had a good relationship with her manager and although she didn't yet trust me, she trusted her manager's judgment. She had witnessed many traumas in her career.

Vicarious trauma can show up as an intense preoccupation with a story you were exposed to. It can change your view of the world and your sense of safety within it. *"VT is a cumulative process: we are not referring to the most difficult story you ever heard; we are talking about the thousands of stories you don't even remember hearing. Where do those stories go at the end of your day?"*[7] The negative effects may manifest as sleep difficulties, intrusive images and avoiding situations that remind you of the traumatic experience in the story.

There was one particular experience that kept Martha stuck. She suffered with intrusive thoughts, not so much about the incident itself or the gory details, but that the attending physician had left her alone to cope with the

---

6    Mathieu, Françoise. The Compassion Fatigue Workbook. Routledge Taylor & Francis Group 2012, pg 9

7    Mathieu, Françoise. The Compassion Fatigue Workbook. Routledge Taylor & Francis Group 2012, pg 9

traumatized family afterwards. She had probably supported many families dealing with trauma in her day-to-day activities, but on that day, the accumulation of all her traumatic experiences got to her. We all have our limits—there comes a point where what we hear and see becomes too much and our hearts and mind shut down to protect us.

Martha came to the conclusion that it would be helpful to have a chat with the attending physician. She felt the need to have her memory validated by him and let him know how difficult it can be to be left alone with family members after traumatic events have taken place. It was also helpful that she had a good relationship with the physician making it easier to carry out that conversation. Of course, Martha knew that physicians cannot be there to offer support all the time, but she learned a valuable lesson after that conversation that encouraged her to ask for support when she recognizes she needs it.

Another way that fatigue can be felt in the workplace is called "burnout."

*"Burnout is a term that has been widely used to describe the physical and emotional exhaustion that workers can experience when they have low job satisfaction and feel powerless and overwhelmed at work."*[8]

Another of my clients, "Jim," was a lab technician. He was recently separated and had two young children. His

---

8    Mathieu, Françoise. The Compassion Fatigue Workbook. Routledge Taylor & Francis Group 2012, pg 10

supervisor was not empathic to his situation. He needed Jim to complete the tasks of his job with no question. The supervisor demanded increased hours and was not able to give Jim the flexibility that he wanted to meet the demands he was facing at home. Jim began to realize that his unhappiness was not just at home, but also that the tasks of his job were not satisfying him anymore and this was leading to frustration. The relationships at work and at home were affecting his ability to function. Jim's feelings of burnout—his feelings of powerless and hopelessness—began to erode him physically and emotionally and he didn't feel good about himself. With awareness he came to see he was no longer satisfied with his job and he began to remember parts of his past that he had forgotten he once enjoyed. He eventually decided that it was time to take a risk and step into a different direction he'd been thinking about for many years and change his job.

## The adapted stress response

The stress response has evolved as a way for our bodies to respond to the dangers we perceive in our environment. You don't get to choose how you will react under stress: your body decides what's best for you instinctively as a way to survive. The stress response is an involuntary reaction, protecting you the best way it can, based on what has been learned, experienced and stored from your life experiences.

Here is my interpretation of the four reactions to a perceived stressor:

- **Fight:** Your body decides to take a stance and challenge the danger head on. Your system organizes itself so the blood flow is greater in the muscles of your upper body to create enough energy to defend yourself and to help you to survive.

- **Flight:** Your body decides that the danger is too threatening and you need to get away, so the blood flow increases to your legs to allow you to run to safety.

- **Freeze:** The body decides that the danger is so frightening that your system shuts down to protect you and you become immobile temporarily.

- **Faint:** The body is so overwhelmed with fear that your system collapses, feigning death as a way to survive.

Peter A. Levine, PhD, has spent forty-five years studying and treating stress and trauma. He holds doctorate degrees in medical biophysics from the University of California at Berkeley, and in psychology from International College, Los Angeles. He is the developer of Somatic Experiencing®, a naturalistic approach to healing trauma. In *Waking the Tiger*, Dr. Levine writes about healing trauma. He talks about how some animals, when threatened, pretend to be dead, and then when the danger passes, they pick themselves up, give themselves a shake, and carry on.

This is somewhat oversimplified, but we humans have a similar ability to pick ourselves up and dust ourselves off. Unfortunately, even after we shake it off, our bodies may respond whenever a trigger reoccurs, even though the event is over. The memory and the emotions may stay with us long after the danger has passed.

## Signs and symptoms of stress

Stress can show up physically in our bodies as headaches, teeth grinding, heart palpitations and general muscle tension. I know that I hold my stress in my shoulders and when I become aware that my shoulders have risen up to my ears, I can, with that awareness, breathe, stretch or move to help my body feel more relaxed and comfortable. Some people experience gastrointestinal issues, backache, insomnia or fatigue. Becoming aware of where and how we hold our stress allows us to spot the first signs that something needs our attention.

Some people, when under stress, react with anger or irritability. Some people have learned to defend themselves this way and it may have worked well for them during childhood and while growing up. However, as adults, this behaviour may no longer be acceptable, particularly in the workplace. When I worked as an occupational health nurse, I heard about an angry surgeon who threw a surgical instrument in the operating room. It hit the hand of a nurse, causing her an injury that required sutures.

In a similar way, we often see patients under stress getting angry at the nurse or health care provider for not meeting their needs in a timely fashion or when their pain is overwhelming.

When a situation gets out of control, it can impair our ability to make decisions. Unchecked stress can result in people taking greater risks with their health, as seen when nurses turn to drugs and alcohol as a way to soothe themselves. And health workers may start to avoid patient contact as a way to avoid that stress.

These ineffective patterns of coping can increase problems with personal relationships and decrease the quality of work relationships. Co-workers often notice such behaviour long before a person acknowledges for themselves that there is a problem.

Covering up, supporting and enabling a co-worker's behaviour is common. Confronting is rare. I would like to think we are at a time in nursing when we can support one another and ask, "Are you okay?" – knowing that it's okay to not be okay.

**If you recognize co-workers not being themselves, asking and caring about their mental well-being gives them a strong message of support. It could really help that individual getting help sooner rather than later.** Reducing the time to treatment could make a significant difference, not only for the health and well-being of the individual, their co-workers and family, but also to the organization's bottom line. Ongoing support can be powerful in influencing the outcome—whether an employee returns to work or not. An added benefit, which is on all managers' minds, is to reduce the cost of medical absences and the associated costs of replacement and training to keep their departments running.

Nurses who have been on the receiving end of harassment and bullying experience other symptoms of stress. They begin feeling like outcasts and they may start to doubt their own abilities and negative self-talk may creep in, eroding their confidence. They may distance themselves from their usual hangouts to prevent further harassment and they may feel guilty that they are not performing as well as they once did. Along with that comes the fear of losing their job if they don't make changes. Increased worry and anxiety can lead to distancing, sadness and crying spells.

When stressors continue, they can affect spiritual and emotional health. This can happen for nurses experiencing ongoing harassment and bullying, and can also affect nurses who are not satisfied in their current positions and roles. The signs of emotional stress can include feelings of hopelessness and a lack of meaning or purpose. This can be a very lonely place to be, feeling isolated and unsupported, and experiencing the loss of self-esteem or self-worth.

## The role of cortisol in stress

Under emotional pressure, we either hold our breath or breathe shallowly. Shallow breathing gives the brain the message that we are dying and sends stress hormones to support the lack of oxygen. The hormone cortisol is released from the adrenal glands in response to stress. When stress goes up, brain growth (neurogenesis) goes down. (As an aside, the birth of new neurons was discovered back in 1970 by a young scientist named Michael Kaplan, who found it in the brains of rats. Up until then it was thought that we were born with a certain number of brain cells and that they started dying off over time. It took till 1990s for science to accept that new neurons could grow in people, too.) In fact, chronic stress can shrink the brain, making it hard to learn new information or even to retain the information you already have.

Cortisol is also the culprit for weight gain, particularly around the middle. For female nurses going through menopause, that's a cruel compounding factor to the difficulty of losing weight as we age.

### Neuroregulation

Circulating stress hormones are released in response to events that occur intrinsically or extrinsic to the individual's experience and the length of time they remain in the body varies from person to person. Different sources quote that these stress hormones may last anywhere from fifteen minutes to several hours depending on how you react to a given situation. What affects one person may not necessarily affect another. I have witnessed some of my clients under stress such that their emotions are not regulated even days after experiencing a perceived traumatic event. Their constant thoughts are replaying, causing worry and creating a barrage of stress. This causes them to experience "brain fog" and they may have difficulty making productive decisions.

**We can bring ourselves into a more relaxed and balanced state when we become aware of our stressors, know our needs, pay attention and act upon them.**

Learning to regulate our emotions through breathing can interrupt the negative feelings and thoughts we have in stressful moments. Paying attention to the natural rhythms of our bodies, recognizing when stressors affect us and shifting our attention to focus on the breath will all help us cope better under stress.

Dr. Diane Poole Heller, a somatic attachment and trauma expert, says, *"When your nervous system is regulated, that's the amygdala whispering, you are not in your fear. Your threat response is extinguishing into exploratory orienting, openness, and curiosity. You feel safe! The whole way you feel in the world, and the whole way you act in the world is very different."*[9]

---

9   https://dianepooleheller.com/

## Checking in on your own stress symptoms

There are many different ways individuals respond under stress and we need to learn to recognize our own symptoms. Symptoms are our bodies' way of communicating: are you paying attention?

Next, we need to learn how to release the tension that creates our symptoms. We have physical needs, too - do we shut them down to serve others first? This may feel like our training or a badge of honour. Either way, this self-denial does not serve us well for the work we do as caregivers.

The caregiver workload is here to stay. Can we change our ability of how to handle it?

## How to SHIFT

When you recognize that moment of stress: Stop and just breathe.

It's the simplest exercise and yet it's so hard to be mindful and to become present to yourself and your own needs. Let's encourage each other to breathe when under stress and remind each other when we recognize what's going on. There are many teachings on breathing from yoga and Pilates training. Here's a technique, named coherent breathing, that I learned from Tara Brach, a world-renowned leader in meditation and spiritual teaching in her online course, "Awakening your fearless heart." [10]

---

10   (https://www.tarabrach.com/courses/)

## Coherent breathing

The stress response mobilizes the sympathetic nervous system and results in a flood of adrenaline and cortisol. Coherent breathing slows the sympathetic nervous system. It also allows the parasympathetic system to slow down the breath and bring it back into your natural easy flow of air in and out. It's called "coherent breathing," because there is an equal count for the in-breath and out-breath. I like this technique for its simplicity. It is easy to remember and, under stress, you need to be able to remember easy ways to get relief. The best response has been observed when you count to five on the in-breath, hold your breath for a count off two, and count to five on the out-breath. Research posted on January 16, 2019 says that this is the optimal number to calm down the nervous system.[11]

Breathe in deeply and breathe out slowly. Place your hand on your belly to feel it rise and fall; this tells you that you are getting the air in deeply and effectively. Repeat this cycle at least three times and then allow your breath to resume its own natural rhythm.

## When coherent breathing is not enough

When you are experiencing more than the average day-to-day stress (at a level that could lead to a panic attack),

---

11   (https://www.psychologytoday.com/
ca/blog/psychiatry-the-people/201901/
how-yoga-and-breathing-help-the-brain-unwind)

coherent breathing may not be sufficient to bring you back into equilibrium. Try taking shorter in-breaths and prolonged out-breaths. This will help the parasympathetic nervous system calm you more quickly. Purse your lips and imagine that you are blowing through a straw: nice and slow. Peter Levine, PhD, recommends saying the word "Voooooooooooo" for as long as your out-breath will take you, and keep repeating this until you feel calmer.[12]

---

12 Peter Levine PhD stress reduced breathing technique demonstrated by Katie Brauer, https://www.youtube.com/watch?v=6DeB_CGtOJM

# CHAPTER 3:
# Shifting stress from your mind

*The Serenity Prayer*
*God grant me the serenity to accept the things I cannot change*
*The courage to change the things I can*
*and the wisdom to know the difference*

*—Theologian Reinhold Niebur (1892-1971)*

This poem reminds me that when I'm feeling stressed, I can ask myself: *Where is it coming from and can I do something about it? Do I have the courage to change the things I can and let my inner wisdom help me accept the things I cannot change? Most importantly, do I have the wisdom to know the difference?*

Daniel Amen, author of the book, *Change Your Brain, Change Your Life*, tells a funny story about discovering that he had an ant infestation in his home. He said it began with just a couple of ants crawling around, which was no big deal. Then a few more joined the party and before he knew it, the ants were everywhere. They had taken over his kitchen and he needed an expert to get rid of them.

He compared this to the thoughts that we have in our heads. One or two negative thoughts are no big deal; add a few more and we can still cope and carry on. But if we are inundated with them, we need to stop and have an intervention because they won't go away on their own. He named these ANTs our "Automatic Negative Thoughts."

**Learning not to believe every thought we have is a skill that is critical to ending suffering.**

"ANTs pop up in your brain automatically, seemingly out of nowhere, and when left unchallenged, they bite, nibble, torture and infest your mind," says Dr. Amen.

Thoughts affect your mood and your behaviour and unaddressed ANTs can destroy your day.

\* \* \*

Kim was suffering from an "ANT" infestation (Automatic Negative Thoughts) when she was asked to take an extra shift. It was flu season and many of her colleagues had called in sick. She really didn't want to go in and risk picking up the virus to bring home to her family. She hadn't had the flu vaccine herself—she had been avoiding the occupational health nurses roaming in the hallways with the "vaccine cart." But she needed the extra cash for Christmas, so she decided to accept the shift, anyway.

On the drive in, her thoughts turned to getting sick. Was it worth it for the few extra gifts she could buy? *I've done my full-time hours.* She thought she was probably just an extra body and nobody would care if she showed up or not. She considered turning around to go home and then calling back to let them know she remembered an appointment.

As she drove, the ANTs struck: Kim wondered if "chatty Cathy" was on this shift—that would drive her insane. And what about Stella? She would hound her for a donation for some community event she was organizing. She wondered if the violent patient in 201 was still there-she didn't want that assignment! There were endless what-if's circulating in her mind and she felt quite nauseous by the time she arrived. The ANTs had taken over.

When Kim arrived, she was met with smiles and hugs of appreciation for making the effort to support her team in crisis. The manager was bringing in pizza for lunch as a way to say thank-you for all the extra hours put in. Kim thought, *Oh! This isn't going to be a bad day after all.*

* * *

If we deal with small stresses when they occur, we can avoid and prevent the ANT infestation. A good way we can do this is to be mindful of our negative self-talk.

Dr. Rick Hanson, a psychologist, and the author of *Hardwiring Happiness*,[13] says that we have a negative bias for good reason. He suggests that it came from our primitive hunter-gatherer days. Keeping a look out for danger in the world was how we survived. If humans were not alert and anxious and watching for danger to keep themselves safe, they could end up as the lion's dinner. He goes on to say that some people are blessed with "positivity genes," while others are not. It can be difficult if "positivity genes" aren't in excess in your lineage, but the good news is that positivity can be developed when you are motivated to change.

Dr. Hanson says that positive thoughts are like water going through a sieve whereas negative thoughts are like Velcro tape and they stick in our minds. To plug the holes in our sieves, we need to be mindful of the moments that bring us joy, peace and laughter. To notice a caring gesture and respond with a kind regard or thought can help rewire our thinking over time.

Another way is to use our photos. They're great for stimulating positive memories because we can repeat a good experience by looking at the pictures. We can post them in visible places or share them with friends and family on social media.

---

13    Hanson, Rick, PhD Hardwiring Happiness: The New Brain Science of Contentment, Calm and Confidence. Penguin Random House, 2013

## How do we develop negative thinking habits?

When we arrive as babies and even before we develop language, we are taking in information from the outside world: through our eyes when we see our caregivers and colours and shapes; through our noses when we smell the environment and foods that are given to us; through our ears when we hear voices and other noises; and through our mouths when we suck and when we take in different textures, tastes and temperatures. And we also receive information through our skin, through the pressure of the contact we receive.

Do we feel Safe? Secure? Loved? The presence or absence, or the less-than-loving experience of any of these sensations is information. The brain doesn't discern between good or bad. It doesn't know what it doesn't know. We develop our beliefs and our understanding of the world based on our unique experiences.

The information we take in travels through networks of neurons to the parts of the brain that store the sensations we have felt, heard, seen, smelled and tasted. Over time, the stored information turns into patterns of learning and emotions from the time of the experience, ready for a recall. The brain doesn't respond in linear time, so if a present-day experience triggers a memory from the past, it will respond as if the experience is happening right now.

The emotional experience in the brain is stored in the amygdala, a small almond-shaped part of the brain that retains all of our emotional responses. The amygdala regulates emotions and plays a part in how memories are stored and this storage is influenced by stress hormones.

Other parts of the brain that are involved in memory are the hippocampus associated with episodic memory as well as recognition. The cerebellum is said to store procedural memory– for example, tying your shoe laces and playing the piano. Pre-verbal or unconscious memory exists in what is called "implicit memory," which develops from our conception until about eighteen months of age. This implicit memory keeps records of very early events that we are not consciously aware of or able to access. This is in contrast to the memories that we can recall, which are part of "explicit memory."[14]

## Where do beliefs come from?

A belief is an acceptance that a statement is true or that something exists because we were told so, according to Michael Tomasello, a professor of psychology and neuroscience at Duke University.[15] He goes on to say that "since we experience the external world entirely through our senses, we find it hard to accept that these perceptions are sometimes subjectively distorted and that they are not necessarily reliable experiences of objective reality.

---

14    Vanderkolk, Dr. Bessel. *The Body Keeps the Score: Brain, Mind, and Body in the Healing of Trauma* (2014) explains this concept in more detail.

15    https://www.pnas.org/content/115/34/8466

To predict and explain the behavior of others, one must understand that their actions are determined not by reality but by their beliefs about reality. Classically, children come to understand beliefs, including false beliefs, at about four or five years of age.

Michael Tomasello's insights, gleaned from nearly three decades of research on great apes and children, help answer a fundamental question: How do humans differ from other great apes in cognition and sociality? Tomasello has applied a comparative and developmental approach toward seeking answers. His studies on the psychological processes of social cognition, social learning, cooperation and communication shed light on human uniqueness as well as on the cognitive abilities of our closest ape relatives." Tomasello, who is emeritus director of the Max Planck Institute for Evolutionary Anthropology, was elected to the National Academy of Sciences in 2017.

By the time children reach the age to attend school they have created a template of their personal belief system. It is scary to think that each of us is operating on a belief system created by our four- or five-year-old selves! There is good reason to challenge some of the thoughts we have as adults.

"Another important factor accounting for resistance to changing our beliefs is the way our beliefs are so often intertwined with how we define ourselves as people. Indeed, beliefs are associated with a part of the brain integrally involved in self-representation. We want to feel that we are consistent, with our behavior aligning with our beliefs. We constantly try to rationalize our own actions and beliefs, and try to preserve a consistent self-image. It's embarrassing and quite often costly in a variety of ways to admit that we are fundamentally wrong."[16]

Some of the common beliefs that could be adding to your stress are:

> *I am not good enough*
> *I am not worthy*
> *No one ever listens to me*
> *I am a failure*
> *I do not deserve love, health, success or money*
> *People do not like me*
> *I have to be perfect, or else*
> *I am unlovable*

Along with common beliefs, there are also common cognitive distortions that can cloud our assessment of what we are experiencing and that can make a situation seem worse than it really is.

### All-or-nothing thinking

This can also be called "black and white thinking." These include unhelpful patterns like using terms like "always," "never," or "forever" in situations that are not absolute.

---

16    http://www.skilledatlife.com/
how-beliefs-are-formed-and-how-to-change-them/

Kim may say, "I'm always booked to work on all of the statutory holidays." She feels the schedule is unreasonable and that she is being treated unfairly. And she may carry that mood into her day.

It may be true that she has worked all of the holidays over the last year. Then again, looking for evidence to support this thinking, she may discover that she actually has had some of those days off. What we choose to believe, and make meaning of, is up to each of us individually. We have a choice about how we tell our story to ourselves. Here are some more negative patterns we can fall into.

### Overgeneralization

After having a negative experience, we then expect that negative outcome to keep repeating.

For example, Rhonda asked her co-worker for help lifting a patient and when she didn't get the help she needed, she decided that it was not worth asking others for help.

Her co-worker answered in a brusque tone, "I'm too busy", and Rhonda felt isolated and alone, and now she expects this to happen every time she asks for help. Maintaining this negative distortion will keep Rhonda isolated from collaborating with her peers and may leave her dissatisfied with her career choice in the long run. If she could reflect on her practice, she may realize that not all staff members treat her this way. There have probably been other times when she has been supported. Being aware of this overgeneralization and balancing it with more rational thinking will help her stop this pattern of thinking and behaving.

If, in fact, Rhonda is being rejected every time she asks for help, she needs to face this reality and do something about it. There are safety standards related to lifting. Taking responsibility involves opening a courageous conversation to report and change the culture, for her own safety, and for the safety of her patients and colleagues. (More about this in a later chapter.)

## Mental Filter

When we have a mental filter, we get trapped in selective thinking—often remembering only negative events. Imagine a nurse, Amy, who is stressed about her workload of patients on a particular work day: she goes home very tired, still thinking about all the demands. There may have been some lovely words from a patient or co-workers on her performance, or thank-you's she didn't hear because her mental filter was not allowing them through.

To break this pattern, at the end of her shift, Amy could take the time to look for three positive things she saw, did or heard during her day. This can shift her selective thinking and allow her to remember her day differently.

## Disqualifying the positive

You've met this nurse (let's call her Chris)—no matter what positive comment you make to her, she gives an excuse and doesn't accept the compliment. She does not feel that she deserves your positive feedback. For example, if you say, "I really liked the way you supported that mother with her fussy baby today," Chris may reply, "It wasn't anything."

She doesn't respond with any recognition of the compliment she just received, or even a simple "Thanks."

## Jumping to negative conclusions

Joyce decides that if she calls in sick, no one will believe she is really sick. She has no evidence to support this but she has seen the reactions of other nurses when staff members don't show up for their shift.

This is, in fact, a difficult situation because the help is needed on shift but Joyce does not want to spread her infection to patients and others. It's a judgment call and all nurses need to decide for themselves when they don't feel well enough to work or there is a risk of infecting others. Joyce is tempted to report to work even with a fever, for example, just to prove to co-workers that she is not well. But then she will end up going home early and this is not helpful for anyone.

Joyce needs to accept that there may be judgments concerning her decision to call in sick, but how she addresses these will be key, not only to her own recovery, but also to her ongoing relationships with her co-workers.

## Emotional reasoning

Stephanie is quick to tell herself that she's a terrible care-giver for not giving a dying patient the time he needed at his bedside. She feels awful for not being there as much or as often as he wanted, even though, at the same time, she was dealing with a code and a family in distress. On another day, she may have been dealing with her own emotional turmoil because of a recent family crisis. The feelings and the facts get mixed up and this negative thinking can affect her self-esteem—she feels that she has fallen short.

## Setting unrealistic expectations

Charlotte often talks about having to get all of her assigned patients bathed, up and dressed before breakfast and she considers herself a failure if she doesn't manage it. Nurses like Charlotte are heading for trouble. Setting impossible demands, not just on herself, but also on the patient who may be hurried in a way that upsets them, is not helpful and could cause setbacks to the patient's recovery.

Some good strategies for Charlotte include setting realistic goals, resetting goals and letting go of the rigid control of the day's tasks.

## Labeling and mislabeling

Ava just caught herself charting in the wrong patient record. She was working on many tasks, she was distracted and was not present with the task at hand. When she catches her mistake, Ava calls herself stupid. This internal name calling and labelling of herself as stupid could reinforce a belief she holds about herself. Mistakes happen but how we repair them and how we treat others who have made mistakes is important. It all works out better if we can look at the mistake in a positive way and learn from it. This can give nurses confidence to work together and develop relationships that are supportive in their teams.

### Catastrophizing

Olivia tends to magnify an event or comment into a life and death situation—blowing it up to the extreme. For example, if she sees a child walking around in the patient's room, she may then imagine the walking turning into running and an accident waiting to happen. A fall on the concrete floor could cause a head injury, haemorrhage and possible death if he doesn't stop right now!

Good advice for Olivia might be to slow down her thought processes and analyze whether there is, in fact, a dangerous incident waiting to happen. Reigning in her out of control mind to bring herself back to the present moment, breathing, centering herself and feeling more grounded. After reflecting, her response to the situation may be different—and she may find more peace of mind.

## Personalization

When something goes wrong in a patient's treatment plan and the outcomes are not what she thought they would be, Emma starts to second guess herself and she wonders what she could have done to prevent the event even if she was not the cause. Emma's mind churned, *If only I'd checked on him sooner, would I have picked up the change in status and called for help earlier?*

When difficult situations happen, it is helpful to reach out and ask for support or connect to the resources your employer offers. In some settings, learning debriefs and emotional debriefs—bringing staff together to reflect on their experiences together—are very helpful.

Learning debriefs are valuable as a quality practice to prevent future mistakes. The investigation can pinpoint the breakdown of a process or a product used, for example. An emotional debrief allows team members to support one another in a non-judgemental way, fostering collaboration and resiliency. These help nurses and other health care providers not to feel alone in their decision-making and can provide reassurance, support and learning.

Cognitive Behaviour Therapy (CBT) was developed by Dr. Aaron T. Beck, MD, in the 1960s, and is considered the gold standard for shifting thoughts. His daughter,

Judith S. Beck, PhD, wrote *Cognitive Therapy–Basics and Beyond* in 1995. I also recommend *Mind over Mood,* written by Christine A. Padesky with Dennis Greenberger. This book is full of examples and worksheets on how to take a negative thought or core belief about yourself and transform it through a series of questions. This process can help you reframe a cognitive distortion you may be having into a more acceptable way to see and accept yourself. Both books could be extremely helpful for any health care professional wanting to work on their own self-care and personal growth.

## How to SHIFT: Practice changing your thoughts

You can take a step toward self-empowerment by challenging your automatic thoughts and not accepting them as true. You *can* change your thoughts. The first step is to be aware of your thoughts.

Let's suppose, for example, that Kim thinks she is not good enough.

She can start by examining the evidence to support that statement. Looking at the scene of a particular event may bring up the thought that she is not good enough. Naming the not good enough feeling allows a narrative to unfold and a witnessing of some past hurt to resurface. With this conscious intention and providing compassionate kind self-talk, it's possible to shift this thought. It is important for Kim not to cloud the event with lots of stories from the past but remain focused on this one event. Suppose, for example, that she didn't get to her patient's room in a timely manner because she was attending to another patient whose needs were a higher priority. She starts to feel down. A familiar pattern happens in her body whenever she thinks about this. Kim starts to have more negative thoughts: *Nothing is going right today*. Her mood begins to change and then a co-worker may hear Kim sigh as she passes her in the hall. The nurse hears Kim muttering to herself, "I can't be in two places at the same time."

Kim believes that she is not good enough because she cannot always attend to all her work when it's required, but that is an impossible standard to set. Nurses must constantly prioritize their work with the ever-changing demands on any given day.

Kim can feel better by looking at her thought, *I'm not good enough*, and saying to herself, "I am doing the best I can." She may also say, "I am responding to my patients' needs as I can, and I'm doing it safely."

You can change your thinking over time by reframing the thought from, "I'm not good enough" to *"I am enough,"* and by practicing shifting that thought every time the negative one comes up. With practice Kim can uplift and soothe herself whenever she gets overwhelmed by this negative thought of not being good enough.

Consider keeping a notebook. Note any cognitive distortions like the ones described above that you recognize in yourself. In later chapters, I will offer more tools to help in transforming those thoughts into more helpful ways of thinking.

Through my own work, I was able to identify where some of my stressors originated. In the next chapter, I will share more about my story and the conflicts I experienced and some of the tools I have learned to shift my own stress.

# CHAPTER 4:
# Find your voice with courageous conversation

*As we let our own light shine, we unconsciously
give other people permission to do the same.*

—*Marianne Williamson*

The hierarchical establishment in England taught nurses
in training to speak only when spoken to which reinforced
my authoritarian childhood. Finding my voice so that I
can speak up for myself and ask for what I need has been
an ongoing journey for me. Growing up in an environment
where my father, a physician, saw his patients in our home,
I had to learn to be quiet and obedient. I adapted to listening, unable to be boisterous and loud as a child. I became
sensitive to the sounds all around me. While I initially
viewed my upbringing– to be seen and not heard– as a

negative, it has served me well to be able to listen to my client's needs in the work that did as a nurse and the work that I do now as a therapist. As my confidence developed, and with further education, I became better able to sit and counsel people that were in distress.

I experienced a breakthrough moment during an intensive week during my psychotherapist training. The exercise was to remember a personal loss and share, in writing, any memories, unsaid words, heartfelt sorrow and insights inspired by remembering. I chose to write a letter to my mother, even though she had been dead for twenty-five years, to finally tell her how her passivity and submissiveness made me angry. I vowed that I would never be like her, but that's who I had become anyway. I shared how I was breaking that pattern with new thoughts and relationships. I was also able to tell her what I appreciated about her: the compassion and caring she taught me. The difficulty of finding our voices takes honesty and courage.

Conflict is difficult for most of us. I don't know anyone who has learned to "handle conflict well" while growing up. My ability to write a loving letter to my mother is a demonstration that change is possible. I was able to shift from being passive, through behaving in passive–aggressive ways, to being assertive. And I like what Carl Jung, the Swiss psychologist, said–and I'm paraphrasing here– "And when you get through to the other side, you will be more beautiful, authentic and empowered."

When you achieve a desired outcome like that—breaking a pattern of learning—it brings satisfaction and confidence not only into your life, but also into your children's lives, too. Breaking the generational patterns of trauma is healing on so many levels. I believe this is what Marianne Williamson, American author, politician and activist, meant by "shining your own light." You become a role model for others to find their light too, stepping aside from the darkness and leading to that source of light within.

## Changing our brains (and our responses)

There is solid evidence that ongoing neurogenesis (birth of nerve cells) occurs in the adult brain—and such growth can persist well into old age. If you look around at the surroundings you are in right now and observe the items in sight– a chair, a painting, a clock– they all began by somebody having a thought. It is important to have awareness of the thoughts in our minds. They will come and go and what we choose to focus on can be nurtured and can grow like seeds in a garden. Then ask if these thoughts are supporting you to lead the life you want or to be the person you want to be? Our subconscious thought patterns operate like a program in our mind and those thoughts affect our moods and our behaviour. Imagine an iceberg in the ocean, the tip that we can see above the water line represents the conscious thoughts we have and this is only five percent. The iceberg below the water represents our subconscious thoughts at ninety five percent. No wonder it is so hard to change when we don't have conscious awareness of what's underneath that could be holding us back, blocking our behaviours, sabotaging our efforts.

Remember the old vinyl music records? I think of the grooves in the old records as an analogy of how holding on to all the messages, memories and experiences of our lives get deeply etched as pathways in our brains to create neural "grooves." Living from those familiar patterns, whether we like them or not, remains until we consciously become aware that we'd like to make a change. When we introduce a new thought or idea, it may compete with the established "grooves." But if the new thought or idea grows and is used more than the old thought or idea, it creates a new pathway in the brain. Donald Hebb[17], a Canadian psychologist, intuited in 1949 that if two neurons are active at the same time, the synapses between them are strengthened. He coined the phrase, "Neurons that fire together, wire together." Thus, a new response is created and the old pathway falls away. That old term comes to mind for muscle memory also, "If you don't use it, you lose it."

When we are under stress, however, our old default responses may come up and this can be discouraging when we are trying to change a habit. Just know that it's part of the brain's survival response (the primitive reptilian

---

17    https://thebrain.mcgill.ca/flash/i/i_07/i_07_cl/i_07_cl_tra/i_07_cl_tra.
html

brain taking over), protecting you the best way it can. The new behaviour, which is just beginning to register in the brain, using the new pathway, can easily be taken off-line. It will come back once the stressor is removed and we can continue to remind ourselves to nurture the new behaviour once again.

* * *

On top of everything else, Kim is trying to lose weight. She has just discovered that her eating trigger is loneliness. She was raised by busy parents who were developing their business and came home late every night. After school, there was no one to greet her, welcome her home or listen to her talk about her day. That's when she started eating as a way to comfort herself and she probably wasn't even aware that that was what she was doing. Kim realized, after years of yoyo dieting from her teens and into adulthood, that she didn't want to live this way anymore.

She has been working on making healthier choices and things went well for a while. But every now and then a family disruption comes up and Kim starts feeling very lonely again. This takes her straight back to her old patterns for comfort. The new behaviour she has been nurturing is hijacked by her response to the familiar stressors.

With awareness and acceptance, Kim will be able to recognize her reactions and return to her healthier choices, strengthening her preferred behaviours and encouraging the new pathways until they are established as her new default response.

* * *

Dr. Dan Siegel, a clinical professor of psychiatry at the UCLA School of Medicine, has developed an excellent model using his wrist and hand to show the evolution of the brain and how it responds under stress. He says that our brain has evolved over time and has three parts to it. Make a fist with your thumb inside your fingers to help you visualize the following explanation. He demonstrates by holding up his hand saying that the wrist and base of the hand represents the brainstem (the reptilian part of the brain). This part we have in common with reptiles. All the basic functions of survival including breathing, heart rate, release of hormones, cells dividing and growing and sexual urges are all autonomic functions of our bodies that are controlled by the brainstem. The next part to develop was the limbic system, represented by the middle of the palm. Dr. Siegel uses his thumb, crossing over into his palm, to represent the amygdala, the part of the brain where the emotional memories are housed. The limbic system is where the fear response ("fight or flight") comes from when your system feels under threat. Then, using his fingers to wrap forward around the thumb, he portrays this as the newest part of the brain, called the neocortex. The fingers touching into the limbic system represent that all parts are connected. The neocortex is the largest part of the brain, about two thirds of the entire brain, and this is what separates us from reptiles. The neocortex contains our executive functioning abilities—the ability to make decisions, rationalize and be creative and all the wonderful things our brains do.

But under stress, we literally "flip our lids." The fingers wrapped around the thumb (amygdala) are released and the rational, thinking brain goes offline, leaving us foggy, indecisive and unable to think straight or to learn. The older part of the brain hijacks the newer part. Cortisol and adrenaline flood into our systems—this once short-term survival response to stress has become a chronic way of responding to the challenges of the 21st century living.

## Know your triggers

The "fight or flight" response was very useful in cavemen days—it allowed us to run from a hungry lion—but now the stress could be the red light in traffic when you're running late or it could be having to work short-staffed again. It could be that we feel sick and want to go home early but we are afraid of retribution. Or our patient or co-worker says something that offends us—it could be any number of things. Our response is the same.

The nervous system feels attacked—under threat—and it wants to protect you. The best way to combat this stress response is, first of all, to be aware of what is triggering us and secondly, to find a way to soothe ourselves. Then we need to keep practising the soothing routine until our sense of control returns. The goal is to get the neocortex back on-line again. This is called *self-regulation* and is an important skill to learn for use when we get upset.

Breathing, grounding, meditating, shifting thoughts, shifting position, tapping (an evidence-based stress reduction technique I will share later), being compassionate with ourselves as we change and having a touch resource (more about this in the next chapter) are all helpful ways to bring us back from an unwanted stress response.

Often, when we are under stress, our conversations can go off track, too, and it's easy to see why.

## The SHIFT process

SHIFT is a five-step process I that I use in my practice to help people go from an unwanted reaction to a planned response.

The SHIFT acronym stands for:

Sensations

Happening

Inhale

Focus

Track the transformation

## Step 1: Sensations

Stop and recognize the *Sensations* in your body. Scan your body and notice the sensations you feel when under stress. This is an important first step toward awareness. Before you react as you normally would: Stop. Picture a STOP sign or some other image that helps you to pause when you realize that you have been triggered. Triggering is experiencing a body sensation like tightness in your jaw, tension in your shoulders or back, a knot in your stomach, palpitations, sweating, tightness in your throat or holding your breath. On that first signal, slow down or even stop what you are doing. Can you name the sensation you are experiencing? By naming the sensation or the emotion, you can stay focused and interrupt or stop the negative thought patterns that usually come along with this experience. Often, naming the sensation can tame it.

## Step 2: Happening

Observe. Look around and survey the scene as in any emergency situation. If it's safe to do so, you can decide to act or not act. What is happening? Maybe it's an internal sensation that was triggered by a person or event? Can you check what is happening inside yourself, or something outside, that just got your attention? This is easier if you close your eyes and shut out all distracting external stimuli. Check your self-talk and your thoughts—how do you perceive what's happening in this moment? Who said what to trigger you? Did you hear a particular sound or word? Did you see someone or something? Did you smell something or taste something that you responded to? Was it a touch that your body reacted to? Get curious about the way your body reacts and when it reacts. You may start to see patterns that help you link the reactions you have to certain stressors.

## Step 3: Inhale

The conscious intention to breathe allows oxygen to get to your brain and interrupts the action that made you react. Breathe slowly, in and out, using the coherent breathing described earlier—breathe in for a count of five and breathe out for a count of five. When you have mastered slowing down your reactions and slowing down the response pathway in your brain that allows your rational thinking brain to stay online. You now have another way forward to calming your mind and your body.

## Step 4: Focus

In the nursing process, it is important in any assessment to evaluate the situation and consider the outcomes of your action or non-action. Change the focus from your *thinking* to how you are *feeling*. Take your attention away from your head and put it on your heart. Put your focus on your intention, on the response or outcome you most desire. Focus to get clarity on your next action or to soothe a negative thought. This will bring self-compassion to this stressful moment. Now that your mind is quieter, practice listening to your inner voice; listening to your intuition. Trust your inner wisdom to guide you in the direction that's right for you. Focus on your feelings. Ask yourself what the sensation you are feeling needs? What do you need? Can you give yourself what you need in this moment or plan to arrange to meet your needs later?

**Step 5: Track your transformation**

Slow down and become aware of the situation in the present moment. Take that familiar negative reaction and turn it toward a more positive response. Consider tracking your efforts by noting what's helpful in making your planned transition and what's not. If you experience tension in your shoulders under stress, for example, then you can use this as a marker to track as you practice the SHIFT steps.

Changing behaviour takes time and effort and tracking your progress can help keep you motivated, especially when you see successful small steps towards the change you want to make.

As you practice these steps more fluidly, they will transform your stress from a reactionary behaviour to a more mindful response. This slowing down from reaction to response can take just a few seconds. It could save a life – for example, if you are reacting to road rage. It could save your job if you are reacting in anger. It could save your dignity if you react with judgement. It could save a relationship. Practice using this SHIFT process whenever you get overwhelmed and notice what happens when you do. Repeated practice of this exercise allows re-patterning of your brain to override your reactions. It's well worth the effort to save any relationship and particularly the relationship you have with yourself.

## Become aware of non-verbal cues

Continuing to have conversations after we are in an aroused or dysregulated state does not usually have a good outcome for either party. Staying calm helps de-escalate our reactions along with those of family members, patients, doctors and co-workers and is a necessary skill in today's charged and fast-paced work environment.

We observe and react to the non-verbal parts of conversations, if not consciously, then on a subconscious level. Eye contact and prosody—that is, the patterns of speech you use and the intonation of your voice—play a big part in communication along with gestures and your body language. For some, this non-verbal form of communication is focused on more than the words themselves.

* * *

Kim remembers asking Sue for support one day. Sue said, "Sure," but at the same time, she rolled her eyes.

Kim felt uneasy, because the words and body language were incongruent.

\* \* \*

The difficulty in communication is that we assume that our message has been interpreted in the way we sent it out. Professor Albert Mehrabian, Professor Emeritus of Psychology at UCLA, developed a new communication model in the mid-to-late 1960s. Dr. Mehrabian has become best known for his publications on the relative importance of verbal and nonverbal messages. His findings have been misquoted and misinterpreted in human communication seminars worldwide to become known as the "7%-38%-55% Rule."[18] This refers to the relative impact of words, tone of voice and body language when speaking. His research was based on the feeling of communication and the finding that words alone convey far less feeling than the combination of tone of voice and body language. But his work has been misinterpreted as saying that ninety-three percent of communication is body language and only seven percent words.

The formula (7/38/55 percent) was established for situations where there was incongruence between words and expression– that is, where the words did not match the facial expressions. In Dr. Mehrabian's research, specifically,

---

18    https://www.toolshero.com/communication-skills/
communication-model-mehrabian/

people tended to believe the expression they saw, not the words spoken.

## Courageous conversations

Remember that a difficult conversation, well planned, along with an invitation to understand and relate to another person, sets the tone for resolution. If you need to sleep on the problem, discuss it first with trusted others who will listen carefully. Then allow yourself to think about it.

Who says you must have the conversation right now, just because it was requested? If you are not ready for that discussion, then assert yourself by saying so, and request a delay to help you prepare. You can frame a delay in response to the other person as a beneficial thing that will help you both come to a better resolution because the response you give will be better thought-out and reasoned.

If you can share your perspective of the problem from the other person's point of view and they can name the problem as they see it, you will be able to come to a mutual understanding and then together you will be able to resolve the issue.

I have seen many interpersonal situations in which the problem is not identified or understood clearly. When there is no validation of the emotional turmoil caused by a person's problem– maybe owing to not enough time, the changeover of management, individual manager style or even the inability of the person to express themselves under the stress of an investigation—may leave them feeling more distressed. This leads to greater complexity in resolving an issue when conflicts do occur.

What I hear from my clients is that the lack of acknowledgement or validation of events or problems leaves a perception of unresolved misunderstandings and this makes them feel devalued. When Human Resources representatives or managers deal with conflict between co-workers, for example, and don't take the time to listen and acknowledge their perspective, this can give the perception to the employee that they haven't been heard or supported.

We each need to find our own voice when it comes to conflict. What crosses a line for one person may not necessarily be something that feels inappropriate to others. We each need to develop our own relationships within our teams. When expressing distress or asking for a change from someone else, it helps to use "I" statements, rather than "You" statements.

For example, if you enter a "Staff Only" break room and find your co-workers in conversation and they aren't speaking English, you could say, "Hey, I'd really like to join in the conversation but I don't understand your language. Can we speak English?" or whatever language is the cultural norm for that workplace.

Another example could be instead of avoiding a co-worker who normally hasn't supported you in taking a break, you could say, "I feel unsupported when I ask you to cover me for a break. The next time, could we arrange break times at the beginning of our shift, so I can plan my patient care accordingly?"

Here's an example of conflict between a nurse and doctor (I'll call them Mary and Dr. Joe) and a courageous conversation. Mary was new on the team, and it seemed that every time she voiced her observations of Dr. Joe's patient, he interrupted her. She felt shut down. She approached him privately and told him how she felt. She reminded Dr. Joe that she was not a new grad. Mary said that she knew her job well and that she was sharing her knowledge of his patient to support the plan of care, which she reminded him, was part of her job. Dr. Joe apologized and agreed he had cut her off and taken out his frustration from another part of his day on her. Their relationship was repaired and they have since gone on to respect each other's roles and to talk to each other in a way that fosters mutual respect.

The courage she showed in approaching the doctor and sharing her point of view is admirable and helps him to understand her position. It can be a challenging conversation to have but being courageous can result in much improved outcomes for everyone involved.

**Conflict can provide an opportunity for personal growth and satisfaction. Understanding a situation from another's point of view can bring about needed change.**

Again, courageous conversations can foster relationships and can help teams face the challenges of changes in process, mergers and usual practice and policy with communication that is encouraging, understanding and shows mutual respect.

If it does not feel safe in approaching the person with whom you've been in conflict then look at the resources available to help you. Most workplaces have policies on conflict and when approaching a co-worker face-to-face is not feasible, a list of alternative resources may be provided. These may include clinical leaders, managers, Human Resources or Occupational Health Departments. Employee Assistance Programs (EAP) are often available to provide off-site services for employees and their families, too.

Unresolved conflict and the uncomfortable emotions we feel around it can affect the energy we bring to work with us every day. Every person has a certain energy level or "fuel in the tank" and when it's empty, it doesn't take much to start responding in negative ways. "Having a full tank" means that the employee is more likely to get through a shift without feeling depleted.

\* \* \*

When Kim is feeling the stress of her workload and she begins to feel flat during her work day, that is a cue that her coping strategies are not working and she needs to figure out other habits that will help her get through her eight- or twelve-hour day.

\* \* \*

## Perspective and intention

Individuals bring a variety of circumstances to their work. There could be a new baby in the house causing sleepless nights; they could be dealing with a sick or teething infant; they could be dealing with ill parents or other family members; they could be struggling with relationship problems; or maybe they are planning a wedding or vacation. Divorce, separation and menopause also complicate our work lives. The nurse, herself, may be ill or grieving the death of a loved one. She has to take care of herself or maybe take care of someone else in the family in a moment of crisis.

No one can prevent the stressors in life or the workload. That is out of our control but we can work with a different perspective about the job demands and manage the energy that we bring into the workplace.

All of these circumstances can be stressful and learning techniques to handle the stress can help ease our minds. Knowing that we have tools if and when we need them really helps.

It starts with an intention.

\* \* \*

Kim got to bed later than she should have—she just couldn't resist staying up to watch her favourite TV show—and she woke up feeling grumpy. She got up and fed and walked the dog. When she got back, her husband announced that he had invited friends for dinner on one of her days off—she was so looking forward to having some quiet time. She didn't have time to discuss it though, because she had to raise her voice to get her teenage kids up and moving. Joe didn't have his project finished and he blamed her for not helping when she said she would. It was late and she had to leave to get to work on time.

Her stress had started to build before she even left the house. On the way to work, someone cut her off and she yelled at them. She arrived for her shift and learned that two staff members had called in sick with GI symptoms. She felt depleted before her shift even began.

Now, let's rewind and start again...

Kim knew she couldn't stay up, so she recorded her TV show to watch on her day off. Then she took a long relaxing bath with her favourite aromatherapy oil—its calming effect always helped her sleep.

She awoke rested the next morning and delegated her daughter Kristie to feed and walk the dog. Her husband told her that he wanted to invite friends over and she replied, "Sure, can we talk about it later tonight?" She decided that Joe's unfinished project was not her responsibility—he had had weeks to finish it. In a calm voice, she told him that he needed to talk to the teacher to find out what his options were.

She got into the car, rested and confident, and when the other driver cut her off, she was able to calmly let it go, recognizing it was the other persons poor driving skills, not hers. Not allowing someone else's behaviour to affect her mood or day she could continue to listen to her favourite station on the radio.

## Energy and communication

Each of us has an energy body and we feel this intuitively when we are in each other's presence. It's called Prana in yoga and ancient India. The Chinese call it Chi or Ki. I think that in nursing during the intimacy of what we experience in caring for our patients and others, we hone these skills and become sensitive to the needs of others. Sometimes we read the cues correctly and attune to others and meet their needs and other times we misinterpret the cues and make mistakes. I have come to understand this energy misinterpretation as being a projection of our needs (consciously or subconsciously) onto others and this is something we need to be aware of. Knowing the boundary between your energy and another's when you work in close proximity to each other is useful. The way to know if you are absorbing the other's energy is different for everyone—it's the way it shows up for you. Sometimes it can feel like a physical tension or an emotional charge and you are unclear of where it's coming from. It can be good to ask yourself, "Is this my stuff or theirs?"; "Is this about me or about them"? If your mood was clear before contact with this person, then it's probably not your stuff.

Your own self-care practices will determine how your available energy resources will be in supporting you as you go through your day. We are continually expanding our energy with good experiences and contracting it with not-so-good ones. If our energy is low before we start work, it won't take much before we start overreacting to things we would normally be able to cope with.

For nurses interested in learning more about energy psychology, I recommend reading material created by psychologist David Feinstein, PhD, and his wife Donna Eden. She was born seeing energy in herself and others and she believes that all children have this ability. But because most parents don't see the flow of energies as adults, there is no language or discussion to promote learning more about ourselves in this way. She has had the good fortune to continue seeing energy throughout her life and has written extensively with the support of her husband, David. Her wisdom and knowledge of healing techniques is invaluable and her enormously big heart prompts her to share this with the world. Donna Eden states there are nine energy systems from the aura surrounding our physical body to our internal systems called Meridian Pathways, Chakras, Radiant Circuits, Triple warmer, the Electric Circuits, the Grid, the Celtic Weave and the Five Rhythms. These are the basis for a five-minute energy exercise routine she has created.[19] This routine is said to establish positive "energy

---

19    https://edenenergymedicine.com/donnas-daily-energy-routine/

habits" in your body which strengthen your immune system, help you gain energy, feel younger and relieve pain. I want to briefly mention the Chakra system here.

## The Chakra system

Chakra comes from the Sanskrit, *cakra,* which means "wheel." According to yoga traditions, a chakra is one of seven points in the human body, each responsible for a specific "spoke" of physiological function and emotional experience. Yoga and meditation are a means of keeping all of the body's chakras open to the circulation of spiritual energy which is essential for health and emotional well-being. Each chakra represents the energy of the physical body it surrounds and if it is congested or blocked, or when the chakras are not aligned, it can affect the health of your physical body, just as the lack of blood flow from the coronary arteries to the muscle of the heart can cause angina or a heart attack.

The root chakra sits at the base of your spine. It is connected to the earth and represents nurture, nourishment, stability, grounding and survival. Imagine the colour red at the base of your spine as a spinning vortex going in a clockwise direction, seen in front as well as behind your spine.

Continue in the same manner going up the spine and repeating the visualization for the second chakra, called the sacral chakra, which sits between the base of your spine and below your belly button. The colour of this second chakra is orange. This one is connected to your sexuality and relationships to others, including your relationship to money. The third is yellow, and lies in the solar plexus. This is your power centre and is connected to the relationship you have with yourself—your self-confidence, self-esteem and self-worth. The fourth chakra is in the mid-chest area and can have either a pink or green colour. The heart is connected to all of your emotions. This is the middle of the system. The three chakras below are earth-related and the three above are more spiritually-connected. The fifth is at the throat area and is connected to your creativity and expression. Its colour is a sky blue. The sixth chakra is between the eyebrows and is for guiding your intuition. Imagine it being the colour indigo. Lastly, the seventh chakra is purple and it sits four to six inches above your head. This is a connection to the higher self, higher power and spiritual guide.

There are many beautiful exercises to balance the energy of your chakras. Try this one: visualize the colours of the chakras and imagine where each one sits along your spine. The optimal position is to see it aligned with your spine. When it is off balance you may see the chakra spinning in front or behind your spine. The goal is to visually arrange the chakras going up your spine in a straight line from root to above your crown; that will bring them into balance and optimize the health and function of your body. So, for each chakra check where you see or sense the chakra and bring it into alignment with your spine.

The chakras all have different sounds and further meanings in addition to their colours. If you are interested in further study, you may want to read *Charge: The Vital Key to Healing your Life, your Chakras and your Relationships* by Judith Anodea, PhD.[20]

## Alternative therapies

I know many nurses who practice Reiki and Healing Touch Therapy to promote healing for themselves and, with consent, on their patients, too. These eastern techniques are beginning to be more accepted in western medicine. Both of these offer a healing modality based on the principle that the therapist can channel energy into the patient by means of touch to activate the natural healing processes of the patient's body and restore physical and emotional well-being.

## How to SHIFT: Zip-up exercise

With permission, I'm sharing one of the energy exercises from Donna Eden's five-minute energy exercise here. This one is called the "Zip Up." By connecting the central and governing meridian pathways in your body, the energy your hands create during this exercise protects your energy

---

20    Published by Hay House, April 2018

from "leaking out" during the day. By creating this invisible energy barrier, you protect your own energy from becoming depleted as you care for your patients. The central energy pathway goes from your pubic bone straight up the front of your body to below your lower lip and the governing pathway goes from the tailbone, or coccyx, up the back of your body, over your head and extends to above your top lip.

Place the fingertips of both hands together and trace the central pathway three times from bottom to top like you are "zipping up." Then, reach your hands behind your back and trace the fingertips up your back along the governing pathway and over your head to the top of your upper lip once. If you can't reach and you are unable to trace all the way up your back, you can pull up an imaginary line with your hands until you get over your head.

I teach these exercises to people who are looking for more natural ways to help themselves align with their own innate energy and healing. This is especially useful in the environment of a hospital where illness and disease surround you and where protecting caregivers' energy from being depleted is essential to maintaining wellbeing. Again, the purpose of this exercise is to "zip" in your energy, inhibiting leakage and preventing people taking your energy.

If you feel any anxiety, irritation or frustration before your day starts it's a good idea to release this before zipping up. A quick exercise if needed is to make fists with both hands and swing them up and crossing them above your head. Then swinging your hands back down forcefully with sound "whoosh" as you open up your fingers and let go of all that you want to release. Repeat several times till you feel your energy has shifted.

I find this so important to share with my clients. Sick patients can "suck the energy" right out of their caregivers. You may have experienced that feeling—maybe you didn't understand why you felt so drained afterwards. The "zip up" is also protecting your chakra system.

Another way to think about your energy, as you go from room to room caring for your patients, is that you could potentially be absorbing their negative energy and accumulating its effects during your shift. When you feel drained from a procedure or interaction, take either your left or right hand to the level of your upper abdomen (the solar plexus area) and push it away from your body. Cutting this energy off between one patient and another—with intention—and subtly as you leave one bedside and go to another, protects your own energy from being depleted. Without awareness of the build-up of negative interactions (energy exchanges) during the course of your day could potentially affect the next unsuspecting patient. The difference could leave you with a normal tiredness, rather than an exhausted feeling.

Another practice you can try with the intention of leaving any accumulated negative energy from your work day and not taking it home with you—pick a point of exit. This may be placing your hands on a desk or chair at the end of your shift or walking through a doorway or exiting the parking lot. Wherever you choose the exit to be, notice the spot and pause long enough to say something like this to yourself, "And I choose to leave any accumulated stress in my mind and body as I leave for the day that is not beneficial to my well-being." This intentional act can protect your energy and prevent taking negative energy home with you. Getting tired is unavoidable. I'm attempting to give you choices to protect what you have decided where and what to expend your energy on. Daily choices will either fill you up or drain you more.

# CHAPTER 5:
# Shifting Stress Through the Body

*The real act of discovery consists not in finding
new lands but in seeing with new eyes.*

—*Marcel Proust*

I had been working at the hospital for about a year when one day, out of the blue, our clinical educator asked me to do an in-service presentation to orientate new staff to our organization. She wanted me to do it the next day. She had a prior commitment and was not able to present the orientation herself and so she was looking for someone to do it for her.

I felt the blood drain from my body. I froze in that moment and sheer panic took over. She must have seen the look of terror and disconnection on my face as she asked, "Are you okay?"

"No" I responded, "I'm not really good at public speaking. Is there anyone else available?"

I was grateful and relieved to hear that she did find another staff member who was willing to give the presentation but I started wondering why I was so defensive. A part of me had shut down to protect myself from doing something I didn't want to do. I really would have liked to support her but a much bigger part of me was too scared at the thought of standing on a stage. Maybe it was time for me to challenge my fear of public speaking. Part of me knew that holding back from this request was also holding me back from reaching my potential. I wanted to help staff cope with their stressors, but I was stressed, myself, in my own world. How could I put myself out there for others when I hadn't resolved my own fear? How was I going to be an assertive, confident woman behaving this way?

I had discovered that my passivity was a learned behaviour from my Mum and I no longer wanted to be this way. I had to learn to shift from being passive to assertive. Me just saying in my mind that's what I wanted to do didn't make it happen and so I went searching for ways to shift myself to the assertive confident woman I wanted to be.

## Emotional Freedom Techniques (EFT)

I remember very clearly a week at work in the summer of 2007 when we got survey results reported by HR from staff about their work experience. It stated that sixty eight percent of staff felt stressed in any given day. To think that that proportion of staff were experiencing stress at work was disturbing to me and I felt that familiar desire to do something about it– I wanted to make a difference. That very weekend, I was travelling to go to the cottage with my husband but we were not able to get across the lake on Friday evening due to an unexpected storm. We decided to wait it out in a motel for the night. There I discovered EFT from a pamphlet sitting on a shelf in the motel lobby. I left a message for the local therapist to contact me and she did. We spent a couple of hours together and I eagerly went home to learn more, deciding that this was that quick and easy to learn technique that could help the staff with the stressors at work. I loved that EFT had the ability to clear emotional distress and I signed up to begin my certification. I thought that if I wanted to be able to teach this technique to others, then I needed to experience the benefits for myself.

I was required to practice on a hundred people over the next year before taking my level one exam with the founder, Gary Craig, in September of 2009.

Earlier in the spring of 2009, I saw an opportunity to do some hands-on training on abundance and the law of attraction. I was thinking about my problem with public speaking. I felt hesitant but I was willing to try anything to overcome my fear of speaking in public and learning to see myself as abundant would mean I would have to release my fears. And so it was that I found myself in the beautiful coastal town of Long Beach, New York, attending a trauma workshop with Master EFT coach and author Carol Look.

The conference room had a view overlooking the Atlantic Ocean. It was a warm, friendly atmosphere with about fifty women and there were two support workers who would help us through the session.

Carol got right into the work during that first morning. The woman beside me was grieving the death of her teenage daughter the year before in a motor vehicle accident. She stood up bravely at the front of the room and told her story, tears streaming down her face. While telling her story, she used the EFT tapping technique. The tears stopped and she was able to unfold lovely memories about her daughter. Calmness came over her body as she returned to her seat. Another person got up and told her story and then several with similar stories of sexual abuse got up.

I was unable to focus on what these other participants were saying. I was focused on my internal voice. It was saying, *What if I'm expected to go up there, too? Why did I sign up to do this workshop? Why can't I live with myself and just accept I don't have to ever speak up?* I continued to be inside my head and felt a numbness throughout my body.

During coffee break, I went to the bathroom and I broke down crying—uncontrollable sobbing. The more I tried to pull myself together, the more my whole body shook.

What was happening to me? I did not experience any of the horrendous things the other women were talking about that morning and yet my body was remembering something that triggered my reaction.

I left the bathroom, and walked back to the room where the session was being held. My legs were barely moving. I was trying to go forward but my legs felt like they wouldn't move. Was it fear? I got half-way in and broke down again. I was so embarrassed at the way I was behaving. My mask totally fell off in front of this group of strangers. Carol saw me and asked me if I was okay. She saw that I was not and arranged for Rick, one of her support workers, to help me. He sat me down and with the palms of both his hands moving in a rhythmic fashion, he tapped the insides and outsides of my calves as I sat there, unable to talk. I was not able to tell him why I was so upset because part of me didn't really know. After about ten minutes, which seemed like an eternity to me, I was calm enough to hear his voice asking me to breathe. I took some air into my lungs and took my seat for the next part of the day.

I sat in shock at what had just happened. I didn't understand why I had reacted that way. I knew that, before the weekend was over, I would have to challenge myself to put my hand up and take a turn to work with Carol, too.

I tossed and turned all that night about what I was going to say when it was my turn to speak. Even just introducing myself to the workshop group seemed nearly impossible for me. My mind shut down and I had difficulty hearing others say their names because I was so focused on not being able to say mine. I repeated inside my head, "My name is Vij. I am a nurse..." By the time it was my turn, I felt so overwhelmed about getting the words out that I had palpitations and I felt anxious and sick in the pit of my stomach.

Now I was standing, looking out at a sea of faces, with Carol beside me. I trusted this group; they had made me feel safe by sharing their own pain and suffering. Who was I not to do the same?

Carol started to ask me questions about the first time I remembered being scared to stand up and use my voice.

Well, there were lots of times with my Dad. He was an authoritarian, domineering person and there was no arguing with him. "No earlier memories?" Carol asked gently.

"Yes," I said. I was about seven years old and the whole school had gathered for a talk about fundraising for "Save the Children" in Africa. The teacher asked me to go up on the stage to point out where Africa was on the map. I was sitting cross-legged at the back of the assembly on the floor with the rest of the kids. I walked from the back of this very large room up to the front and up a couple of steps to the stage. The teacher gave me a long wooden stick and asked me to point to Africa on a very large drop-down map of the world. I took the stick and touched somewhere on this map, saying, "I don't know."

I don't remember if the teacher asked me to try again but my anxiety about making a mistake and uncertainty about what would happen next clouded my memory and I landed that heavy pointer stick on a place that obviously was not Africa. I was so surprised when I found myself on that big stage and I didn't know what to expect. When I think back now, it would have been nice to be treated with some kindness or help to move that pointer stick to the correct position to show where Africa was. Instead, the teacher said in front of the whole school that I was wrong. The kids all started to laugh and the teacher asked me to go sit down again.

I walked off the stage with my head down—I didn't want to meet anyone's eyes while they laughed at me. I quietly sat cross-legged at the back of the assembly room again but I don't remember much more after that. The event never came up in conversation with parents, teachers or other students ever again but it was burned into my brain.

Carol worked with my emotions of shame, humiliation and embarrassment—these were all aspects of my fear. This experience taught me that making a mistake in front of a group of people should be avoided at all costs. She helped me understand that, even as an adult, the anticipation of speaking and feeling these emotions was a trigger for my unresolved trauma. The fear came with me into my adult life. As long as it remained buried and unresolved in a part of my implicit (unconscious) memory, I was not able to access it. My fear kept me safe from experiencing more shame, humiliation and embarrassment.

As children, how we associate our thoughts to events is not always rational. It didn't make sense that my brain may have done all that interpreting to protect me from further humiliation, but I was able to use the tapping technique to reach a level of calm in which to reframe my fear successfully.

I rated my emotions on a 0-10 scale (where 0 meant no fear and 10 meant the most fear I'd ever experienced) and my scores all dropped from 8s to 4s in a short time. I was standing there for about half an hour while this unfolded. I was able to see more clearly a part of myself that had good reason to be scared and why I wanted to protect myself from further humiliation by not using my voice.

Also, I remember when my kids were small. They were four little girls having so much fun playing together. I had felt an uneasiness in the pit of my stomach when I heard their prolonged laughter, especially after meals. I called that spike in their energy their "daft half hour." I could only tolerate that pitch for a short time before I had to shut it down. Their laughter was a trigger for me that I was unaware of at the time. When I think back, I feel sad that I was not able to allow that joy into my life. My seven-year-old self's unresolved trauma at being laughed at for a mistake affected so much of my adult life.

I'm happy to report that I don't think any of my girls suffered from being asked to quieten down when they were little. When they get together now they still get boisterous, loud and laugh out loud. The difference is that now I can tolerate it and laugh along with them.

I learned so much about myself that weekend that made sense to me. Once I gained this understanding, I was able to reframe the story I carried of myself and install positive beliefs. I'll talk more about that later.

I went to my room that night so excited to have unravelled a part of my past that had been holding me back—I actually jumped up and down on the bed like a little kid. Then I had a wonderful sleep.

### Performing a body scan

Stress can come from any number of past or current events in your life. One of the best ways to get in touch with how you're holding stress in your body is to scan your body from head to toe.

When I get stressed, I hold it in my shoulders. They tighten and hunch up around my ears, causing pain, and that tells me something needs to shift and change.

Our bodies are always talking to us but are we paying attention to what is important—are we listening? Try this simple exercise. Make sure that all electronic gadgets are turned off so you will be undisturbed for two minutes.

That's all it takes, or even less, when you become more aware of your body.

Close your eyes. Start either at your head or your toes.

I like to start from the top of my head, noticing any tension in my face that I can soften and particularly feeling into my jaw, opening and closing it to relax it more, if needed. Travelling down my neck, I turn my head side to side to notice if there's any tightness to the left or right sides. Then down my shoulders, arms, hands and fingers.

Noticing my breath as I scan my body, I check to see if there's an easy flow going in and out of my lungs. Is there any place I feel stuck, as in holding my breath, or that I'm shallow breathing? These are all signs of stress in the body. The body responds under threat by sending adrenaline and the hormone cortisol to prepare the body for fight, flight, freeze or faint as needed to keep us alive. If I feel any tension, I allow myself to move my arms to get them into a more relaxed position.

Next, I breathe into my belly, relaxing any tension there. As I start to feel more relaxed, the feeling of diminished stress sends a message to my brain that I am safe and this interrupts the stress response.

Lastly, going down my hips, legs, shins, calves, ankles and feet, I notice any areas that are holding tension and breathe into any tight spots.

**Where in your body do you hold your stress? It's so important to recognize the signals your body is giving**

**you. Ignoring that first sensation of stress causes it to get louder and bigger over time. In psychotherapy classes, we learned this saying,
"Whatever you resist, persists."**

Being aware that stress is held in your body—and where you hold it—and noticing the places, events and people that trigger stress are other pieces of your puzzle. The narrative you tell yourself about your life and your experiences can shift and change each time you unpack your memories, a little at a time.

Carol told us that weekend that EFT is based on the Chinese meridian system. This system describes where practitioners insert needles to relieve pain as in acupuncture (acupoints are the end-points of meridian pathways). There are no needles in EFT but we tap with our fingertips (index and middle fingers) on eight end-points to stimulate these meridian pathways we have in our bodies.

We can thank Gary Craig, an engineer from Stamford University, for founding the "basic EFT recipe." He took complex algorithms developed for many physical and mental health conditions that he learned from Dr. Roger Callaghan, a psychologist from the United States, and with his engineering brain created a simple version that addresses common emotions that most people experience.

EFT is an evidence-based stress reduction tool that is effective and easy to learn. I love to teach and empower health care professionals to use this whenever I can.

# EFT - The Basic Recipe[21]

Tap with your fingertips on these eight points on your upper body while talking about an emotional stressor at the same time and you will be able to help put the brakes on the sympathetic nervous system and your stress response. This allows the parasympathetic side to "rest and digest" and calm your nervous system.

For those skeptics who need further evidence, you can look up the EFT research journals, peer reviewed papers and presentations by Dr. Dawson Church[22] and Dr. David Feinstein[23]. There have been more than a hundred peer reviewed papers so far which all support the use of this technique for emotional distress, fear, phobias and trauma. Review the diagram showing the tapping points before reading further. See Appendix B.

## EFT Procedure

## Step 1
You want to get paper and a pen before you start. Then get comfortable in a space with no distractions and take three easy breaths.

---

21    Information on EFT training in Canada https://www.neftti.com/

22    https://www.eftuniverse.com/english/reprinted-academic-articles

23    http://www.innersource.net/em/about/david-feinstein.html

Focus on a situation that has upset you. Next, name the emotion that's associated with the situation you are thinking of. This is called the "target" and it's important to name what you are targeting. The more specific you are will help you get clarity on what that emotion is all about and what it needs in order to let it go. Spend some time writing down all the thoughts that you have around this event and all the reasons you feel the way you do about what happened. There may be a few or many reasons contributing to the way you feel.

Imagine that trees in a forest represent your negative life events. As you clear each negative event, or chop down a tree, a clearing appears. Sometimes clearing a few trees can collapse the whole event without having to chop down the entire forest.

If you have difficulty coming up with anything to work on, think about the following three things to help you identify some blocks or negative beliefs: things that irritate you in others, triggers in any of your relationships or try setting yourself a big goal (like writing a book!) and see what barriers come up for you.

Removing the emotional attachment to an event allows an understanding that can strengthen the core of who you are. By giving your emotions space to move through you, you can allow those suppressed emotions to be released. Understanding and accepting one event at a time and clearing the negative energy that is blocking you can help you create more space for renewed energy that you can use towards the life you want to lead.

## Step 2

Now rate your emotional response using a zero to ten scale, where zero has no intensity and ten is the highest intensity you have ever experienced. Write this number down on your paper. If the intensity is above five, start by tapping about five to seven times at each point, at a speed comfortable for you, while thinking more generally about your emotion; for example, "overwhelm" or "anxiety." Tap so that you can feel the stimulation at each point but you shouldn't feel any pain while doing this.

This helps take the edge off before going further into the story of what's overwhelming you or making you feel anxious—calming your nervous system to allow a gentle release. This helps you maintain focus and prevents the memory from re-traumatizing you.

A note of caution: If you have memories that are traumatic, please don't do this alone. Find a knowledgeable practitioner who can support your healing.

If your intensity number was five or lower, work with a specific event and go through the story in your mind, piece by piece.

## Step 3

Now you are going to create a "set-up statement." This could be something like, "Even though I feel overwhelmed when I think about my job and what I have to get through today, I accept myself and all my feelings."

Some people may have difficulty saying, "I accept myself" so you could substitute, "I want to accept myself" instead.

Say this statement out loud or inside your head three times while at the same moment, tapping on the "Side of the hand" spot—the S of H. (This used to be called the Karate Chop spot in some articles.) Start by using the fingers of one hand to tap on the opposite hand, on the side of your palm, between the pinky finger and the wrist. It doesn't matter which hand; it is a very forgiving process.

## Step 4

This is where you will choose a reminder statement. An example could be "all this overwhelm," or phrases from the list you made listing the reasons why this event made you feel overwhelmed. Repeat the statements while tapping on the following eight acupoints on the body. You can tap five to seven times on each point while saying your reminder statement.

> The **first** point (EB) is at the beginning of the eyebrow. (gallbladder meridian)
>
> The **second** point (SE) is at the side of the eye on the bony part. (bladder meridian)
>
> The **third** point (UE) is under the eye in line with the pupil. (stomach meridian)

The **fourth** point (UN) is under the nose. (governing meridian)

The **fifth** point (Chin) is between the lower lip and chin. (central meridian)

The **sixth** point (CB) is one inch below the collarbone and one inch to the side (K27 meridian). Some people like to make a fist where the spot of a man's necktie would sit and tap there, or use their outstretched hand placed on the upper chest, to tap on the CB area. Try all of the variations and use the one you like best.

The **seventh** point (UA) is located four inches below the armpit on the side of the body where a women's bra band would be or for men in line with the nipple. (spleen meridian)

The **eighth** point (T of H) is on the top of the head. (crown chakra) You can either pat your head or do a little dance around the crown of your head with your fingertips. Again, experiment to find which variation you prefer.

There may be a spot that you respond particularly well to – one that creates a feeling of calm for you. This will become your "go-to" spot to massage when you are under stress.

While tapping the eight points, say your reminder statement—out loud or silently to yourself:

EB – All this overwhelm that I'm feeling today

SE – All this overwhelm for the work I have to face today

UE – All this overwhelm is too much to cope with

UN – All this overwhelm that I'm feeling in my shoulders

Chin – My shoulders are telling me how over-whelmed I feel today.

CB – All this overwhelm that is hard to deal with every day

UA – All this overwhelm that shows up every day

T of H – I'm not sure how much overwhelm I can deal with today

## Step 5

Now take a breath and evaluate how you feel. There may be a thought, an image, a colour or a sensation when you get tuned in to the overwhelm (or the emotion you are working with) and what that means for you.

You can re-rate the intensity on the "overwhelm" you were experiencing. Sometimes the intensity you experience goes up because now you are tuned into your problem. Sometimes the intensity stays the same and at other times it drops to a more manageable level. Keep repeating the eight tapping points—it may take several rounds before you feel a shift to lower numbers. It's really important to validate the negative emotions and allow the expression of thoughts to come out. Sometimes it can take several sessions to deal with all of the reasons—when one set of reasons gets cleared, other aspects can arise. Like peeling the layers of an onion, there is more to discover. As you are checking in after every couple of rounds about your intensity, also check that it is still the same target that you started with. If another targeted emotion surfaces, consider this a new aspect and begin as in step one to name it, step two to give a number to the intensity and step three create a new set-up statement.

I like to get down to an intensity of one or two before starting Step 6.

## Step 6

When the intensity of the emotion you are working on comes down to one or two out of ten or lower you are ready to install a positive or reframing statement.

Create a new set-up statement– a positive one. For the example of feelings of being overwhelmed, your new set-up statement could be: "Even though my job is overwhelming, I choose to face my day with ease and grace."

Repeat the tapping process as above, tuning in again to your feelings of overwhelm, while repeating your new set-up statement:

S of H spot – "Even though my job is overwhelming, I choose to face my day with ease and grace." Repeat three times.

EB – I can choose to find ease and grace in my day.

SE – I can find space to breathe between tasks and accept my day.

UE – Noticing my breathing helps regulate me.

UN – I can choose to support myself with kind self-talk.

Chin – I can let some of this overwhelm go.

CB – I can allow myself to feel more relaxed now.

UA – I am enough.

T of H – I'm doing the best I can, and that's okay.

Take a breath and again check in. Re-rate your number, write this down and check on your body sensations to compare to what they felt like when you started.

Try another round, alternating the negative statements with the positives. You can pick the phrases that speak to you or make up your own.

It's important to use your own words, language and feelings. The words here are just an example to help you find your own. Rather than using variations of your set-up statement, you can repeat the same thought at each point, particularly if you are holding a specific emotional memory.

When you begin to feel calmer, you can step back, reframe your thoughts and emotions and begin to recognize the shift you are feeling. You may notice that your shoulders have dropped. Your breathing maybe more even and relaxed. Your thoughts could now be helpful and focused to activate what you want to do next to function in your day.

Using the EFT practice can release fears, phobias, anxiety, guilt, anger, loss, trauma and other negative emotions and any beliefs that may be limiting you. The Emotional Freedom Techniques can be used for daily stress and even when you don't feel stress, you can use EFT to help support and align your energy—like giving your car a tune-up. EFT can also be used to enhance your creativity and performance. Many basketball and tennis players, dance teams and professional golfers tap before each game and they find it helpful for adjusting their mental and emotional strategy.[24]

## How to SHIFT:    The Personal Peace procedure

List all of the things, people and events that have upset you in the past. Look at each decade of your life and see what pops into your mind: maybe when your third-grade teacher embarrassed you when you cried in front of the class; when dad didn't show up for teacher-parent night; when mom forgot to pick you up after school; when the first boy or girl rejected you.

It's all in there, stored away. After making your list—it could contain a hundred or more events—you can go

---

24    www.eftuniverse.com/sports/
eft-for-sports-other-personal-performance

through the list at your own pace, giving each specific event a rating and tapping until it's clear.

It's an easy technique to do but rather ridiculous to look at, so doing it in public is probably not a good idea! Your fingers go wherever you go, so you can try tapping the sides of your nail beds—these also stimulate acupoints—as an alternative when you are out in public. See the diagram in Appendix B to show you the specific tapping points.

Also, on this diagram you will see two X marks. One on the back of the hand and one on the chest. The one on the back of the hand is the end point or exit point of the energy circuit called Triple Warmer. This circuit not only controls our fight, flight and freeze response but it also impacts the immune system and our ability to manage stress, according to Donna Eden of Eden Medicine. When you place one hand over the X marked over your heart area and tap with your fingers of your other hand on the X marked between the fourth and fifth fingers it will have a calming effect on your nervous system.

Your stress is held in your body and it accumulates with each event unless you actively find ways to release it. When you don't look after your stressors, they affect not only your life but also the lives of those closest to you.

So, I hope this chapter encourages you to do something about your stress whether it's tapping, jogging, baking or singing. Find a way that fits into your schedule and do it.

While jogging or baking provide a temporary release for stress, EFT has been found to have a long-lasting effect on the nervous system and reactions will no longer be experienced as they once were.

# CHAPTER 6:
# Stress and Relationships

*Life is not about waiting for the storms to pass....*
*it's about learning to dance in the rain.*

—*Vivian Greene*

We spend most of our waking hours with our team members and so it's not surprising that we see the best and the worst in each other.

## Interpersonal conflict in the workplace

Kim was involved in an investigation on her unit. A co-worker (Jane) had been accused of disrespectful behaviour towards another nurse (Barb). Kim had witnessed the behaviour and she was named in the formal report. Kim worked with both Jane and Barb. They used to get along but now they were talking behind each other's backs and their friends felt they were being asked to take sides.

Kim was uncomfortable at work when these two were on-shift together, knowing that a conflict would likely arise and Kim didn't like taking sides. The conflict also spilled over to their off-shift activities. Kim would get email invitations from a co-worker and notice that either Jane or Barb was excluded. Invariably someone would tell and tension would rise. Kim didn't want to get involved. It was hard enough to get through a shift while trying to avoid contact with either one and to hear the bad language and put downs of the other, without the added strain of being in the middle of it.

After Kim's manager interviewed her about what she witnessed, her manager told her that by ignoring the bad behaviour that she was allowing it to continue. The manager was helping Kim to assert herself when she witnessed conflict. Kim decided she needed to take a position. She had never seen herself as an enabler before and so she reached out to talk about it with co-workers she trusted. From then on, when either of the warring nurses approached her with negative comments about the other, she told them she no longer wanted to hear about it. She told Jane that, since Barb was not there to defend herself, Kim was not willing to witness the complaint this time. Kim told Jane that she wanted to be professional with both of them. Kim realized that, after this, she would no longer be part of creating toxicity in the team. Kim shared this stance with her co-workers and that they each had to decide how they were going to handle the situation if they got involved in Barb's and Jane's crossfire. In time, both Barb and Jane stopped offering negative comments and Kim was able to engage with them in a more honest and open way. It was really hard to work through this difficult time but Kim was relieved that both women accepted her feedback and agreed to work with her in a professional way.

## Violence in the workplace

Sometimes interpersonal relationships become much worse than the conflict between Barb and Jane. In rare cases, physical violence ensues. You don't expect violence to be part of your work day but the reality is that it does exist. I recalled the following true story about an anaesthetist and a recovery room nurse in the Hotel-Dieu Hospital in Windsor, Ontario, when our team in employee health was asked to create a presentation for staff on workplace violence.

In the following article,[25] journalist Larry Cornies shares what happened in their relationship and its tragic consequences. This story has made nurses more aware that mental health is an issue on both sides of the gurney. With awareness, we have a choice about how we interact with our colleagues, peers and patients. We can reflect on

---

25    Permission given by Larry Cornies, journalist and editor for the London Free Press

what's important as we serve our patients and the energy we bring into our workplace each day, while trying to be the nurses we want to be.

The headline in the London Free Press on Saturday, January 9, 2010, read, "Nurse's killing in workplace spurs changes."

> *"Lori Dupont, 37, was the nurse from Amherstburg who died on the morning of Nov. 12, 2005, inside Hotel-Dieu Grace hospital in Windsor. Her killer was anaesthesiologist Marc Daniel, 50, a physician with whom Dupont had, that spring, ended a tumultuous two-year relationship.*
>
> *An 11-week coroner's inquest was held during the fall of 2007 into the murder and the complex set of circumstances that coalesced around the death.*
>
> *The jury in the Dupont inquest produced 25 recommendations, most of them detailed and multilayered, directed to the Ontario legislature, the Ministry of Health and Long-Term Care, the Ontario Hospital Association, Hotel-Dieu Grace, the Ontario Medical Association, and more than a half-dozen other governing bodies and government agencies.*

*Two of the recommendations included provid-
ing a program that would train all hospital
personnel on workplace violence prevention,
and the other was reporting incidents for
which staff may be liable."*

After the publication of this article, Cornies describes
getting a call from one of Lori DuPont's co-workers. She
was saddened by the details. And she felt that the story
of who Lori Dupont was should be told—she wanted to
honour her memory.

The public is often not aware that caregivers are also
human beings who are dealing with their own struggles in
life while also showing up to care for others. This can be a
difficult balancing act. Most people are not aware of the
kinds of behaviours from co-workers, patients and their
families that staff have to deal with on a daily basis. And the
co-worker support that each colleague provides and relies
on to deal with it makes a difference. This support increases
their resilience and allows them to put on a professional
face masking their hurt and pain and permits them to do
the work they love to do—caring for and supporting others'
return to health.

In the months immediately after Lori Dupont's death,
the article went on to say, *"…staff went from being in denial
and being defensive to being more open."*

Staff in hospitals are starting to accept that violence IS
in our workplace. Although commonly witnessed, that does

not make it okay. It's not acceptable in the community, nor should it be acceptable in health care.

> *"But the single greatest lesson from the Dupont case was the extent to which 'domestic violence can affect someone in the workplace'—that domestic violence and workplace violence aren't separate and discrete problems. One can easily spill over into the other."*

This finding hit home for me, since I have been on the receiving end of domestic violence. I am also happy to write that this was in my first marriage, not my existing one. I was told, back in the 1980s that "You don't bring your baggage to work." We were instructed to "leave it at home." We didn't talk about personal stuff at work; we kept it to ourselves. Talking about other people's business was considered gossip and unprofessional.

Cornies continues:

> *"There was a Neighbours, Friends, and Families workplace-violence prevention program that attracted the attention of the inquest's jury and led to the recommendation of training the staff at Hotel-Dieu Grace, emphasizing the roles neighbours, friends, families, and co-workers can play in violence prevention.*

*To call attention to the positive impact that Lori Dupont's death has had locally, a tree was planted in the memorial garden of the hospital in her memory. In addition, there is now a scholarship in Dupont's name for nurses who wish to pursue additional education. Provincially, Bill 168 was a direct result of this tragic incident in the workplace."*

Bill 168 passed into law in 2009 to amend Ontario's Occupational Health and Safety Act with respect to violence and harassment in the workplace and other matters. Section III of the Occupational Health and Safety Act (OHSA) defines the following:

32.0.1 (1) An employer shall,

(a) prepare a policy with respect to workplace violence;

(b) prepare a policy with respect to workplace harassment; and

(c) review the policies as often as is necessary, but at least annually. 2009, c. 23, s. 3.

**Domestic violence**

32.0.4 If an employer becomes aware, or ought reasonably to be aware, that domestic violence that would likely expose a worker to physical injury may occur in the workplace, the employer shall take every precaution reasonable in the circumstances for the protection of the worker. 2009, c. 23, s. 3.

## Workplace harassment

The OHSA defines workplace harassment as engaging in a course of vexatious comment or conduct against a worker in a workplace that is known or ought reasonably to be known to be unwelcome.

## Workplace violence

The OHSA defines workplace violence as the exercise of physical force by a person against a worker, in a workplace, that causes or could cause physical injury to the worker. It also includes an: attempt to exercise physical force against a worker in a workplace, that could cause physical injury to the worker; and a statement or behaviour that a worker could reasonably interpret as a threat to exercise physical force against the worker, in a workplace, that could cause physical injury to the worker [section 1].

This may include:

- verbally threatening to attack a worker;
- leaving threatening notes or sending threatening e-mails to a workplace;
- shaking a fist in a worker's face;
- wielding a weapon at work;
- hitting or trying to hit a worker;

- throwing an object at a worker;
- sexual violence against a worker;
- kicking an object the worker is standing on such as a ladder; or
- trying to run down a worker using a vehicle or equipment such as a forklift.

The definition of workplace violence is broad enough to include acts that would constitute offences under Canada's Criminal Code.

### Taking a moment to reflect

It has been over a decade since Bill 168 came into effect and the stress of our relationships with each other, with management and with families and patients continues. Bill 168, while providing awareness, did not provide zero tolerance. We can expect conflicts to continue because the very nature of our jobs—caring for a diverse population of patient needs and demands and making life and death decisions—puts us into the eye of conflict.

What has changed is the mandatory programs to educate all staff on these serious topics. It is now law; organizations must create policies and conduct risk assessments of their environments and they must be reviewed annually. By reaching out, reporting and by continuing to implement recommendations, we get better at resolving conflicts and making our workplaces safer for everyone.

It's never too late to voice concerns but you cannot assume that passing information or complaints to an authority figure is going to guarantee resolution—sometimes it doesn't. Senior leaders are also stressed with their workloads and there are a lot of layers between them and the front-line staff.

There are brilliant and passionate people working in healthcare who are making a difference every day. Let's continue to support teams by creating a culture that is trauma informed by the work they do and can recognize and be encouraged to speak up and ask for back up when needed.

Could we reduce the amount of sick leave taken if we felt we could speak up and resolve stressors and challenges as they occur? Changing the relationship with yourself to being assertive confident and compassionate could also help you to be more clearly understood by your managers. It could give managers an opportunity to support you and possibly reduce the fear of retribution.

If you felt safe to speak up and tell management that you couldn't take on another project or cover another shift, would you?

What if it wasn't considered weak to say "No," but just human– an indication that you need recovery time so that you can get re-energized for getting back into the work again?

Showing our vulnerability and our human need to connect and stop for a breather is about self-awareness, self-acceptance and self-compassionate care and should be supported.

## Workplace code of conduct

I work for an organization that offers respectful workplace training that stresses a code of conduct that binds us to work together professionally with dignity and respect and that fosters relationships so that we can support each other.

**When relationships become strained due to misunderstandings, miscommunication, misinterpreting a tone, a look or an action and the problem is not addressed, there is a missed opportunity for repair.**

The impact on us as individuals on the receiving end of incivility and also on witnesses like Kim, from incidents of both overt and covert behaviours, gives rise to emotional, mental, physical and social distress.

Remember, one in five people in Canada will suffer a mental health condition in any given year and half a million Canadians are off work in any given week due to mental health illness. (Mental Health Commission of Canada, MHCC 2010)[26]

When we are not able to repair damaged relationships in the workplace, it starts to have an effect on our

---

26    https://www.mentalhealthcommission.ca/sites/default/files/2016-06/
Investing_in_Mental_Health_FINAL_Version_ENG.pdf

organizations. Nurses leave under these circumstances and rightly so. Who wants to work in an environment of conflict? And those that stay often end up perpetuating the negative culture. Unfortunately, the bottom line is that patient care can also be affected. Mistakes could be made and if patients begin reporting offensive behaviour, mistrust in our healthcare delivery may follow.

We need to find our voices and speak up for the kind of care we want to deliver and the support we need from our co-workers. We need to think about how we can help resolve conflicts as they arise by acting as role models and by engaging in courageous conversations.

## Develop and maintain healthy relationships

It's great when everything is going well and everyone gets along and that's why it's so important to develop good relationships with your peers. When challenges come up, you will be able to deal with them more easily and as you get to know your co-workers better, you will feel more confident in approaching them when difficult situations arise.

The energy you bring into your workplace is important to you, to your teams and to your patients. You know that you cannot change another person, so although this may seem obvious, changing yourself and the way you care for yourself—so that you can bring your best self to work—is your opportunity and responsibility.

I was not raised with a handbook or even a role model that taught me how to handle conflict. Most of us were not. In England years ago, we were encouraged not to get involved in other people's business. We were told to turn away, avoid the conflict and maintain a code of secrecy. Now I'm finding my voice and I'm encouraging people to get involved—to speak up when they witness workplace harassment or violence. Safety is everyone's business and we can no longer turn a blind eye. We can choose to participate and collaborate in finding peaceful solutions. I often will mention Lori Dupont's story whenever I'm in a session about conflict and respectful workplaces. Remembering her death and the introduction of Bill 168 gives us courage to speak up. This helps us break the silence that keeps us isolated and in fear of retribution when we see or experience challenges of our own.

By using the SHIFT process from chapter four whenever you find yourself in a state of conflict, you can help take yourself from a reactionary state to a responsive one. Practicing this exercise over time allows the re-patterning of your brain and you will be able to override your reactions and transform them to reasoned responses. It is well worth the effort.

## H.A.L.T.

This is an acronym referring to never allowing yourself to get Hungry, Angry, Lonely or Tired. Nothing good can come from working from these states. In the nursing world, we can predict that these states will happen if we don't anticipate and plan for them.

When you get upset and angry, there may be good reason but at work it is not acceptable to "shoot your mouth off" under any circumstance. Talk it out with a trusted friend, tap it out (EFT) or learn to meditate to settle and calm your mind. Anger is not a true emotion. Rather, it is a state of mind that is protesting about something, unable to articulate what is needed, much like a child in distress and often there is an underlying feeling of sadness or fear. Anger can fuel you to action and can be a positive force to move you toward a more desirable state. Figure out what your anger is about and do something about it. Your anger is not welcome in the workplace and others may find that you are creating a toxic environment—your co-workers won't want to work with you.

Being lonely is a common state. As human beings, we need social connection, so make it your goal to engage with others. Find a like-minded group to hang out with. Your colleagues may become your friends but they do not have to be. They are your work family and as such, treat them professionally, but you can prevent loneliness with like-minded people outside of work.

If you wake up feeling alone and you need to hear a human voice, consider one of the distress phone services. Also, there are many immigrant families who do not initially have resources to support them. When you are experiencing a challenging time and you have no family and social systems available, life can be difficult. Keep stretching and growing and reaching out until you get to a place you can call home. Volunteering is also a great way to make new friends, to learn new skills and participate in a worthy community cause.

Lastly, do whatever you can to avoid going to work tired. We cannot behave like young children who will fight the urge to go to bed when they feel tired. Give in and get some rest! If this is an ongoing problem for you, it may be good to see your doctor. I will write more about this in shift work stress in chapter eight.

## Boundaries

The lack of boundaries can create a lot of tension in relationships especially when we are unaware of the role they play. We have internal boundaries which help guide decisions about how we will walk in the world. They can protect the way you view the world and define who you are. We are aware of our boundaries through our self-talk, our beliefs and our values. We also have external boundaries that define what we will allow to come at us from the outside world. As we grow and learn, these boundaries can change with us. They are not fixed. They can be influenced—for better or worse—depending on our life experiences and the relationships we keep.

A boundary is a line that separates who you are from who the other person is. Maintaining healthy boundaries is a way to protect yourself. It's important to know your limits—your stuff versus their stuff. It's not easy. Not everyone has developed clear boundaries growing up. Damaged boundaries often show up in dysfunctional family systems that involve physical, sexual or emotional abuse and which have no healthy limits on behaviours.

The following study clearly demonstrated how the health of children can be affected by not developing clear boundaries by dysfunctional parenting. The Adverse Childhood Experience Study (ACE) was conducted by the CDC-Kaiser Permante. The ACE study is one of the largest investigations of childhood abuse and neglect and later-life health and well-being. The study was completed in two stages between 1995 and 1997 in southern California in a predominately middle-class white population. Ten questions were used to survey more than seventeen thousand adults about their childhood experience. The survey asked about physical, sexual and emotional abuse including neglect. The survey also asked whether they had witnessed violence between their parents and whether either of their parents had been incarcerated. In that population, sixty-seven percent of respondents had at least one experience that fell into these categories.

The study showed that adults who had four or more of these experiences went on to have increased health risks compared to adults who did not experience these traumas. You can access the ACE study at the link below to check your own score.[27]

Children first learn to say "No" at around eighteen months of age and not long after that, they start to identify what belongs to them: "It's mine!" These are normal developmental stages for all children. If parents react inappropriately, with "Don't say that," or if they send the child to their room for speaking out, the message to this child is to disown that part of them that is not acceptable. They quickly learn "to be seen and not heard."

Your boundaries may operate properly when interacting with some people but not for others. For example, it may be easy to say "No" to your best friend but difficult to say "No" to a boss asking you to work overtime.

Sometimes when you think you're creating boundaries with others you're really putting up fences and walls to protect yourself. The silent treatment, for example, keeps you isolated, preventing intimacy and making it difficult to deal with issues. Ignoring, avoiding or walking away tells the other person you are not interested in contact with them. This may be how you learned to deal with difficult situations growing up but your walls are interfering with developing healthy relationships. As I learned in school, "Our issues remain in our tissues"–those past painful,

---

27   https://www.npr.org/sections/health-shots/2015/03/02/387007941/
take-the-ace-quiz-and-learn-what-it-does-and-doesnt-mean

unmet or unresolved issues persist, as do the walls, until we become aware of how our behaviours maybe affecting our relationships. Issues from childhood can remain buried but they can also leak out in unwanted behaviours later in life.

## Types of Boundaries

**Physical boundaries** help us to determine the appropriate physical space between ourselves and others. Different cultures prefer different amounts of personal space and we may feel uncomfortable if another's style varies from our own. For example, notice how people re-arrange their positions when they get into an elevator. To determine the appropriate personal space in Western culture, we should be able to have comfortable eye contact with the individual within the allotted space. In addition, physical boundary violations in the workplace could also include hitting, pushing, throwing, shoving and inappropriate touch.

Our physical boundaries give us the right to determine who, when and where others can touch us or get close to us. When we practice self-harming behaviours, physical boundaries may be compromised and this indicates an unhealthy connection to self.

Setting healthy boundaries for ourselves allows us to love and care for our bodies and to know our limits– for example when it comes to food and alcohol intake.

**Sexual boundaries**. It is estimated that forty percent of females and twenty percent of males have had their sexual boundaries violated when they were children. Direct sexual abuse of children includes the fondling of genitals, masturbation, intercourse and exposure to pornography. Indirect sexual abuse includes the lack of sex education by parents. It is a parent's responsibility to protect a child by sharing healthy values and helping a child with their choices. It's not a judgement if a parent doesn't teach their children about sex-topics—they may have not been educated themselves or they may have their own trauma history. Inappropriate sexual behaviour around children or being shamed for being male or female is another kind of sexual abuse. Sexual boundary violations in the workplace include use of inappropriate words, insulting, non-consensual touch or sexual humour that causes embarrassment and shame.

We all have the right to determine how, when, where and with whom we want to be sexual, as long as it is consensual. We can then enjoy sex in a healthy way while also being the gender we most identify with.

**Emotional boundaries** are violated by constant criticism, being raged at or being frequently belittled. In the workplace, this could take the form of name-calling, bullying, angry outbursts or non-verbal actions like eye rolling or dismissive hand-waving.

We have the right to our feelings and we have the right to choose how, when, where and to whom we will express them. In setting healthy emotional boundaries, we learn how to say "No" to others, how to speak up and how to confront others when necessary. We learn the skills to de-escalate, negotiate and compromise during conflict to collaborate and to establish win/win solutions or at least to agree to disagree.

**Spiritual boundaries** are violated when people impose their religious beliefs on others. In the workplace, violations could include co-workers judging you for your beliefs, making fun of your religious-specific attire or making negative comments about your prayer schedule.

When we recover our spiritual boundaries, we learn that it is okay to experiment with different spiritual systems to find one that supports our own view of spirituality.

A good indicator to determine whether your boundaries have been violated requires being in touch with your feelings. When you feel angry, resentful, beaten down, used or overworked, your boundaries have probably been crossed in some way.

When you experience boundary violations, it can negatively affect your ability to collaborate and to care for yourself and others. Boundary violations erode confidence, passion and connection. They increase self-doubt, anxiety and depression—common reasons for absences in our workplaces.

Setting boundaries is really about caring for yourself, realizing you are important, and that your feelings matter. Boundaries help you to stay within your personal power—to know yourself and your limits and then being able to ask for your needs to be met.

Asking doesn't cost anything. Being kind, appreciative, grateful and supportive are qualities that enhance a relationship and worth finding ways to practice. If your ask is related to money, then it may not be as easily resolved with restrictive budgets and competing needs. Your personal values will guide you to have that courageous conversation with a trusted colleague to get support or to get a different perspective on the issue at hand.

## Challenging your "Window of Tolerance"

When you want to shift and to expand and grow, and when you want to have courageous conversations even when you feel overwhelmed, it is helpful to know that everyone has a "window of tolerance."

Imagine upper and lower lines, like the top and bottom of a window. Between these lines is a space that represents your ability to tolerate experiences in your life. In this space, you are flexible and adaptable and you have the ability to hold coherent conversations with great life force energy and stability. Some people may call this your comfort zone.

When babies are born, they have no tolerance for discomfort and they protest loudly with cries. When they are soothed, they learn to expand their window of tolerance and it expands as they learn and grow. When people reach the upper limit of this window, they become challenged and their bodies respond by stimulating the sympathetic nervous system for mobility. When you reach a boundary limit, the stress response is alerted for fight or flight.

Alternatively, when humans reach their lower limit of this window, they are challenged by their parasympathetic nervous system being stimulated for immobility—the stress response here is freeze or faint.

Either response is out of your control when it happens but learning how to respond when faced with challenges may prevent you from reaching your limit. If the challenge is at the top of the window, it's about learning to calm and soothe yourself to find your stable range again or if it's on the bottom of the window, it's about learning to stimulate yourself to get back into the stable range.

Either way, learning to regulate your emotions when you are under stress is very helpful. Work to develop tools that will help you observe your reactions to stressful situations and practice habits that will help you to recover. This will help you stretch and grow each time a challenge comes up. Bouncing back or coping with challenges is called resiliency.

Attachment style

Another piece of the relationship puzzle is knowing your attachment style.

In the 1960s, Dr. John Bolby and Mary Maine, an American psychologist noted for her work on attachment theory, performed what they called the "Strange" experiment.[28] They took thousands of infants aged twelve to eighteen months of age along with their caretaker mothers and they observed the interactions when mother and child were together, after the mother left the room and when she returned to the room. Based on these observations with a stranger present with the child, they developed an attachment theory that categorized children into four categories: Secure, Avoidant, Ambivalent and Disorganized.

Secure children, when left alone, cried when their mother left the room and were easily soothed when she returned. A consistent response of being picked up and comforted by their mother had attached these children securely to their caregivers. These children had learned to trust that their mother would meet their needs. They are likely to grow up with the confidence to trust themselves as well as others in relationships.

Avoidant children continued to play with their toys and did not look up to see where their mother was when she left the room. They also did not react while she was gone or when she returned. These children had already learned that their need for comfort and soothing would not be met by their caregiver. This group of children had learned to soothe themselves and they grew to distrust the world as they grew up. They learned to put up walls to keep

---

28    https://www.psychologytoday.com/
ca/blog/compassion-matters/201307/
how-your-attachment-style-impacts-your-relationship

themselves safe which can create difficulty in relationships and intimacy later on. Their strong independence leads them to a tendency of pushing others away. They are likely to grow up trusting themselves more than others.

Ambivalent or anxious children got upset when their caregiver left the room and they were not easily soothed when their mother returned. These children had received a loving presence but not consistently enough for them to trust that they would be soothed and comforted. Sometimes they got the care they needed and at other times not. Having learned that their mother was inconsistent with their loving attention created anxiety and clinginess. These children became unsure when they might receive loving attention again. They often grow up attending to and focusing on the needs of others and that others have the answers they are looking for to soothe their inner angst. They often grow up trusting others rather than themselves.

Disorganized children reacted with both avoidant and anxious behaviours. They sometimes approached their mother but they would also turn away or fall down. They had learned not to trust this relationship and their behaviour is often seen in children of abusive parents who may have also been using either drugs or alcohol.

Children, as they develop and grow, have a strong desire to go towards a parent(s) for connection, comfort and love. In disorganized attachment, the child also fears the harm that may result in this interaction and pulls away. These children may grow up to repeat these abusive patterns in their own adult relationships.[29]

## The Good News

Everyone is hard-wired for secure attachment so even if your caregivers did not provide these connections for you, other relationships with friends, teachers, peers and partners who are securely attached can help you become secure, too.

What's interesting to note is that more recent research from attachment specialists, such as Dr. Diane Poole-Heller,[30] demonstrate that this original attachment style moves into our adult relationships.

It's helpful to understand that our attachment style continues into adulthood and especially shows itself under stress when we tend to go back to our learned behaviours. The different attachment styles need different kinds of attention when developing trust in our adult relationships—we need to learn to give as well as to receive.

In a healthy relationship, there is an easy flow of give and take, of separation and return, and that helps us feel we are stable and within our window of tolerance.

---

29    https://www.psychologytoday.com/
ca/blog/compassion-matters/201307/
how-your-attachment-style-impacts-your-relationship

30    https://www.dianepooleheller.com

Dr. Sue Johnson, an expert in couple's therapy, recommends that her clients read her book, *Hold Me Tight*.[31] It addresses seven conversations every couple needs to have. She asks "Are you there for me?" Using the word "A.R.E." to expand on a relational concept. "Are you Available, Responsive and Engaged?" What she is saying is: Can I find you when I need you? And when I find you will you respond to my needs? And, also, will you engage with me in a way that supports us?

Applying this idea to our relationships with co-workers sounds like a perfect recipe for secure attachment. There is attachment in all our relationships, not just those with our loved ones. I really want people to stretch this concept into the workplace. Could we ask that of each other at work, "Are you there for me?" Can your co-workers depend on you? Will you be available, responsive and engaged with them? Will you have their backs and will they have yours? Will you trust and grow with them and take risks in your relationships that widen the window of tolerance for all of the challenges you face together?

In healthcare, staff work very closely together and for extended hours. Why not use the same principles that create healthy relationships with loved ones?

---

31   Johnson, Sue, PhD *Hold me Tight: Seven Conversations for a Lifetime of Love*. Little Brown Spark. New York, NY, 2008

## How to SHIFT: Learn your attachment style

Learning your attachment style may be a good way to begin assessing your style in relationships. You can try the short version of the attachment questionnaire available in Appendix C.

How you show up in your workplace is important to patients, to your team and also to you. Without stereotyping, I do wonder whether nurses have common traits that expose them to more stress? That's what I will address in the next chapter.

# CHAPTER 7:
# Do Nurses Share a Common Personality Profile?

*"Be the change you want to see in the world."*

*"As human beings, our greatness lies not so much in being able to remake the world—that is the myth of the atomic age—as in being able to remake ourselves."*

*—Mahatma Gandhi*

Have you ever worked with a nurse who goes out of her way to please everyone? She comes in early, she offers to help above and beyond her own patient load and she stays late, if needed. She is a tough act to follow or aspire to some days, or maybe you don't aspire to be like her at all. She could be the martyr.

I met a nurse recently for counselling. I'll call her Jenny. Jenny told me she was that kind of nurse—she would not only take on her own assignments but when asked to help others with their assignments, she'd drop what she was doing to help them. Sometimes it left her patients in unsafe situations. She understood this but she was still unable to say she was too busy to help in that moment. "I'll be right there," was her response. Others' needs became more important than her own. She had difficulty asking a co-worker to wait and when she left her patient to tend to the care of another, she was left feeling guilty and by the end of each shift, she was exhausted. Doing so much for others, she started to feel she was being used and that made her feel resentful.

This was not comfortable and she was looking for some relief. On the inside, she was suffering. She wore her mask well but her stomach was in knots, she had tension head-aches and she had difficulty sleeping. She knew she was not eating well. She was choosing unhealthy carbs as a way to comfort and soothe herself but she was unable to stop.

Her co-workers had come to know her as this type of nurse, so how could she stop now?

With some work, Jenny realized that, growing up in her family, it was expected that they would always help others without question. She was taught that it was selfish to do otherwise. Jenny needed to understand how this belief was affecting her health and her role in the team and that it was putting her patients at risk. She could see the benefits of changing her thought pattern. Together we worked on shifting her perspective—she needed to take a risk and change the behaviour that was preventing her from being assertive. This change would help relieve her of the stress she was adding to her day.

## Sub-personalities

We all have between five to eight different personalities— there are sides of us that come out in reaction to the people and situations we interact with at work and at home.

For example, I have a fun and playful side when I am with my granddaughter; the student side of me loves to learn; my compassionate side appears when I'm listening to my clients and I'm a controller in my kitchen. I used to have an inner critic but I gave that one an extended leave. I surprised myself by becoming a teacher and author later in life. Who knew that was possible? As I accept more of myself, those personalities that have taken a back seat are now surfacing and I love the creative side that is now available to me. You probably show different sides of yourself to different people—some make you laugh and bring out your silly side, some with whom you have serious talks with and those you want to party with.

Most people know that nurses are caregivers and that they can be perfectionist and controlling in getting their work done, but they can also be the bully or the victim, too.

Carl Gustav Jung, (1875-1961) a Swiss psychiatrist and psychoanalyst, introduced the concept of "archetypes":

basic patterns in human beings that are present in people all over the world. Based on these archetypes is the "psychology of selves." The assumption is that we consist of different "selves"– sub-personalities who each play their own role within the person.

Negative sub-personalities need to be acknowledged for the positive service they have performed before they can be re-integrated into the self. There may be some times in which some of these integrated personalities may still temporarily be required to protect you. In Jenny's case, her caretaking part needed to show up for her patients and she needed this to be accepted by both her internal parts as well as her external team.

**For yourself, try to be aware of your inner personalities so that you can recognize when they begin to sabotage your ability to function in a healthy way.**

There has been more recent work on understanding these parts of ourselves by Richard C. Schwartz, PhD. He took his experience from four decades of family counselling and put it into a model he calls Internal Family Systems (IFS).[32] Schwartz calls these parts "Protectors" in our being that show up as "Managers," to support your socially acceptable behaviours– the ones that get you to work on time, do your banking and organize your day. At work an example of a manager could be that part of you

---

32    https://ifs-institute.com/resources/articles/ internal-family-systems-model-outline

that collaborates with your team as a caregiver or people pleaser. Other protectors, called "Firefighters," are not always so sociably acceptable and these are the ones that drink, gamble, cry, shout and generally stand out when you get in a situation that triggers "Exiles". An example of a firefighter at work could be that part of you that is insensitive to others or sends a put down message to a co-worker. Exiles are wounded younger parts that are hurt, scared and afraid of what's happening in your adult body and may react from that younger state. An example of an exile part showing up at work could be when an authority figure judges you and inside you get triggered from a past event that makes you contract, feel shamed or even start to cry. Whenever the exiles get triggered the protectors jump in with a behaviour that they feel will help you out. So, both types of protectors have been developed in a way to help support your being to survive. Schwartz says there are no bad parts– as they all exist for a reason– and all are welcome and accepted in therapy. This is a reassuring feature to be able to explain to clients. Underneath these parts there is a "Self" that is authentically the true you and uncovering this self can lead you to live a life that you are aligned with. Schwartz calls this a "self to part leadership" relationship: meaning the relationship between the self and all of the parts including the managers, firefighters and exiles. This model can help you negotiate between the different parts of you and turn down the noise in your mind. It can create an inner atmosphere of light, harmony and peace which can bring more confidence, clarity and creativity to your relationships. If you are interested to learn more about this technique, check out the recommended reading in Appendix D at the end of the book.

## Personal experience with sub-personalities

There was a time in my life when I became depressed and unable to cope with the demands of my world—the world I had created and thought I loved. It all came crashing down as I didn't have the awareness of what this "depressed part" was doing FOR me, not TO me. What I understand now, that I didn't back then, is that it protected me from facing the overwhelm of all the responsibility that comes with work and family. During times of overwhelm and dysregulation, my stress response must have had a parasympathetic (i.e. inhibitory) reaction as a way to tolerate the discomfort of what I was experiencing. My system decided to shut down for a period of time as a means of coping. For me, that looked like withdrawal from connecting with family, friends or conversations. And the more the part of me that ignored the stresses showed up, the stronger the "depressed part" got until the energy of attempting to keep it all together was too much and I couldn't handle it anymore.

The other parts of me that loved learning, thinking, planning and being responsible were all angry at this "depressed part." And the "inner critic part" took delight in this ongoing battle! Taking time off turned out to be the best thing that ALL of my parts needed—to take a break, reflect and find some balance between work and family. It was hard to nurture a part of me that could ask for help. This was foreign to me as I considered myself to be a strongly independent person.

By getting quiet and becoming introspective, it is possible to have "conversations" with these different parts inside of us (which, as far-fetched as it sounds, represent ourselves at different ages and stages of life). These parts are often isolated and may get triggered and react in childlike ways that are inappropriate as an adult. For example, if you experienced getting stuck in an elevator or stuck in a closet when you were a young child you may develop claustrophobia.

Therefore, you may avoid stepping into an elevator as an adult to avoid that part of you that makes you feel anxious. If you are unable to avoid this emotional trigger, this younger part may then act out of fear or anxiety. You may be aware of a past incident or not that it is causing this anxiety. Connecting to this part and soothing that scared part is a helpful way to heal a past event that is causing some difficulty in your present-day life.

We can identify and understand our different parts and the roles they can play. It is possible to read and practice this technique but it is more easily supported by a professional therapist qualified in IFS work. At the time I was off, I did not know about this work but I imagine I had to go through a process of negotiation to soothe myself and cope to be able to return to work. I likely had to negotiate with the part of me that wanted to remain independent and do it all by myself. My "non-trusting parts" had to learn to be less defensive with other parts that cared about me and wanted to help me to recover.

There was another part of me– I will call it my "figuring it out part"– that when it got on board, it didn't take long before I was able to understand the needs of the depressed part and to thank it for stopping me functioning for a while so I could pay attention to the decisions that I was making. I began to wake up and see the world I had created for myself and I discovered that I did not like myself very much. I questioned my values and beliefs and started to work towards aligning myself to who I wanted to be. And during this long process, I learned to accept myself, just as I am. This shifted my perspective on how I saw the world and how I handled my problems so that I could face my life and live it more fully.

I'm not suggesting that all depression is as simple as taking a time out. There is a continuum to this condition and every person that I have supported with depression presents with stories as varied as the lives they lead. It's a very personal journey to recovery– depression is treatable.

I encourage my clients to include their physicians in their plan of care to find the right path for themselves.

I have chosen to list a few of the many "sub-personality" mini-profiles here that I recognize from the health care providers I have interacted with over the years. Do you recognize some of your own strengths and weaknesses here? You will find many more sub-personality profiles in Appendix A.

| Sub-personality | Positive function | Negative function |
| --- | --- | --- |
| Caretaker | Nurturing, caring, sees wounds in others | Neglects self, creates victims |
| Comedian | Light-hearted and likeable in social situations | Can be insensitive, and not taking life seriously |
| Controller | Organized and detail oriented | Suffocates others and can create chaos and disappointment |
| Inner critic | Awareness of danger, reality check | Disabling messages and shaming |
| Fixer/Rescuer | Helpful and considerate towards others | Disempowering and neglects their own pain |
| Over-Achiever | Strives for excellence and doesn't give up easily | Easily burns out and often has high demands |
| People pleaser | Diplomatic and finds peaceful solutions | Sells out true self and avoids conflict at all cost |
| Perfectionist | Responsible and gives their best | Rigid and creates victims or conflict |
| Teacher | Shares information, is logical and clear thinking | Rigid, theoretical, and judgmental |

Imagine these different parts existing inside of you. Some days the positive side shows up and on other days, you'll display the negative part and some parts are stronger than others. Imagine all of your sub-personality types riding on a bus: where do they sit and which personality likes to be the driver?

## Our inner critic

We all have an inner critic and, in some people, it's stronger than the other parts of their personality. When I first learned of this concept, I decided that my inner critic was not going to "drive my bus" anymore and so I moved it to a back seat and gave other parts of myself the ability to develop and grow. While the inner critic may have served a useful purpose in the past to keep me safe or protect my weak self-esteem, I came to realize that it was no longer needed to defend my ego.

## Accepting what is

Life would be so much easier if we were able to accept where we are right now and support each other through stressful days. Of course, that's if we lived in an ideal world. We are all at different stages of our growth and development and so being mindful of that, what I can suggest is the following. Let's name what we are feeling and facing so that we can use our collective energy to support each other when work conditions get overwhelming. What if, rather than the sigh and worry and dread of what the next twelve hours will bring, we could acknowledge to each other that it's going to be a tough day? By bringing awareness of what you feel, to accept some of these emotions and give some space for them, could this better support you as you gear up to get through your shift? What would this look like? What may you do differently? Would you offer a gesture of connection, "May you be safe" or give a high five or hug to a co-worker you know well? Could you take a break together to debrief instead of feeling alone and isolated? We are social animals and we need to connect– this is how we survive.

## Our Need for Connection

In his Polyvagal Theory, Stephen Porges[33] explains his concept of the vagus nerve—the "wandering nerve." This theory says that the vagus nerve monitors social connection and safety to engage with others from the day we are born. It gives us messages from these interactions and stores in our memory that which is safe and that which is not.

It's worth taking a moment to review this important development in neuroscience and the huge impact it has on our relationships.

The two branches of the autonomic nervous system (ANS) are the sympathetic nervous system (SNS) that creates mobilization and the parasympathetic nervous system (PNS) from which the dorsal vagus creates immobilization. Porges says there is a third branch, which he calls the ventral vagus. This connects from the gut, through the

---

33   https://www.stephenporges.com

heart and the lungs, to the muscles in the vocal cords. It also runs to our middle ear, our face and head and links into the brain stem—hence the name, the "wandering nerve." Porges believes that this circuit was built for social interaction or engagement, whereas the SNS and PNS were built for defense. He coined the word "neuroception"[34] to describe how neural circuits can distinguish between situations or people that are safe and those that are dangerous or life threatening.

Neuroception explains why a baby coos at a caregiver and cries at a stranger. Our facial expressions, our tone of voice and our gestures all convey messages, including those messages our bodies react to when we are under stress. This is important to know this when we are working with our patients and teams. If our facial expressions, tones of voice, and gestures are not perceived as safe, others will react involuntarily, in an instant. Therefore, we have the ability to put our patients and each other at ease and to make safe connections by how we present ourselves to the world. I knew that keeping calm was important as well as smiling and using a soft voice in interactions but with the new brain science, I now better understand why.

This theory helps me understand and consider the symptoms that a patient could be experiencing as a result of stimulation of the vagus nerve. These could include symptoms from anywhere along the course of the nerve,

---

34   https://eric.ed.gov/?id=EJ938225, May 2004

including upset stomach (stomach), palpitations (heart), difficulty breathing (lungs), trouble with speech (muscles in the vocal cords), impaired hearing (middle ear) and/ or interpretation of danger from a flat facial expression (face). These are all symptoms of a stress response. It could indicate that the patient does not feel safe in that moment. This is a cue for us to offer support and reassurance.

Self-regulation is when we can regulate ourselves, meaning that we can provide a steady, calm emotional response to our external experiences. The self-regulation of one person can influence the regulation of another person when they appear to be upset or what is called "dis-regulated." When we influence another person, this is called "co-regulation". Have you ever come across a person that has just been in an accident or received some bad news? They often become dis-regulated– that's a normal response of our nervous system to trauma or intense stresses. When you offer support, this connection, or co-regulation, can help them to feel better. What if we could recognize our co-workers when they get dis-regulated and offer this same kind of support? It could strengthen a team's ability to cope on difficult shifts. We know we are regulated when our breathing is relaxed and our heart rate is steady. Consider taking your pulse throughout the day and remember to breathe to maintain your own self-regulation.

We also have "mirror neurons" in our brains. This means that when we offer a smile, an openness and a calm demeanour, others can feel it. Have you ever walked down a hall smiling and caught the attention of a stranger walking by? Have you noticed that they often smile back? That's their mirror neurons at work.

## How to SHIFT:    Find your disowned self

Work to accept yourself just the way you are and to make friends with all of the different parts of your personality. When you learn to accept yourself, it may be easier to look at others and all of their personalities with compassion and acceptance, too.

Try the following exercise to shift your perspective of yourself and you may also shift some of the stress and tension you carry. Stress is an inside job. Notice your feelings and own them. We are emotional beings and no apologies are needed.

$$\frac{\text{AWARENESS} + \text{ACCEPTANCE} + \text{ACTION} =}{\text{CHANGE}}$$

This formula was given to me during my training at the Transformational Arts College in Toronto. The origin is unknown, but the College co-founder, Gord Riddell, added that change also takes into consideration a perceived risk. The "letting go to change" isn't possible unless it's safe to do so.

An exercise developed by Hal and Sidra Stone, psychologists in the United States, shows how you can come to know the parts of you that you have disowned.[35] For example, imagine when you were growing up and you liked singing. But every time this part of you emerged it was punished, so you repressed it. When this pattern repeats enough times, you get the message that you are not acceptable or lovable for this behaviour and so you disown it. A disowned self is an energy pattern in your psyche that has been partially or fully excluded from your life.

To find your disowned selves, start by thinking of someone you dislike or, conversely, admire intensely.

Take a piece of paper and divide it into two columns. Think, for example, of a person who really pushes your buttons and whom you really dislike. Now make a list of all the things you don't like about this person in the first column. Then, in the second column, list all the qualities that are opposites of those you listed in the first column. Does the second column look familiar? It should– you've just met yourself with the qualities of who you currently are. The characteristics listed in column one are triggers for you and as you recognize them in others it can make you say, feel and do irrational things. So which person in the two columns is right? The answer is neither—each side has so much to learn from the other. In our daily lives, it is important to recognize that other people may react differently from you in a given situation and it is valuable to learn and to understand how to tolerate these differences in behaviour.

---

35   Hal and Sidra Stone, creators of Voice Dialogue International, 1972
https://voicedialogueinternational.com/index.htm

According to Hal and Sidra Stone, "The people who we hate, judge or have strong negative reactions toward are direct representations of our disowned selves. Conversely, the people who we overvalue emotionally are as well. Here is the Catch 22: in spirituality, we are taught never to judge. Our judge then becomes disowned and we lose this valuable teacher that tells us what is disowned in us and what needs to heal."

I believe, from working in other countries, that despite the fact that our basic human needs are all the same, it is the sharing of cultural differences that helps enrich our lives. I wonder if these differences could be explained from this perspective of disowned parts of ourselves? Those parts that have not been loved and accepted–we have disowned them and we don't want to recognize them but we often judge them in others.

We are usually not conscious of this but our behaviour can be affected in a powerful way by the way others treat us. The universal Golden Rule is succinctly expressed as "Do unto others as you would have them do to you." If this rule is applied to the interaction between two people, there can be great joy in being able to connect with that other person. So, when the safety of connection is experienced with our colleagues, it can lead to more satisfaction and creativity and improved coping.

Rumi, a Persian poet and Sufi mystic (Jalal al-Din Rumi) from the 13th century, understood the different personalities we create and offers a perspective on how to meet and accept yourself, with all your different parts, as they show up in your day and in your life.

### The Guest House
### by Rumi

*This being human is a guest house.*
*Every morning a new arrival.*

*A joy, a depression, a meanness,*
*some momentary awareness comes*
*As an unexpected visitor.*

*Welcome and entertain them all!*
*Even if they're a crowd of sorrows,*
*who violently sweep your house*
*empty of its furniture,*
*still treat each guest honorably.*
*He may be clearing you out*
*for some new delight.*

*The dark thought, the shame, the malice,*
*meet them at the door laughing,*
*and invite them in.*

*Be grateful for whoever comes,*
*because each has been sent*
*as a guide from beyond.*

*— Jalal al-Din Rumi, translation by Coleman*
*Barks (The Essential Rumi)*

# CHAPTER 8:
# Shift work Stress

*If you change the way you look at things,*
*the things you look at change.*

—Dr. Wayne Dyer

Most caregiver positions include shift work, either eight
hours or twelve. I worked on the front lines for about ten
years before realizing that my mind, body and spirit would
not be able to handle the required adjustments in day-to-
day living that shift work demands for the remainder of
my career, so I opted for a management position. I thought
that a steady day shift would better suit my needs and that
of my family, too. With the increased responsibility came
more demands and my day shift started to feel like five
twelve-hour days, with little time for my family or me. After
five years of this, I went on to further studies to specialize
in Occupational Health, which led me back to direct patient

care—and an eight-hour day shift position. I admire the courage, perseverance and dedication of the nurses that remain on the front lines throughout their careers, because it requires some tough decisions as you transition through the life stages.

We each have to make the career choices that suit us. We need to know what our limits are and the amount of sleep we need.

I remember that shift work was not a lot of fun when I was in my twenties, especially when I couldn't go to the pub for a drink with my friends who worked daytime hours only. I also missed family events because my schedule didn't allow me to drive the two hundred miles to the celebrations which were half way across England from where I was working.

In my thirties, when I had my own family in Canada, I actually loved the night shift. It was the only time I could get a solid six hours of sleep. When I worked the day shift, my third ear was always listening throughout the night for the stirring of any of my children who might need my attention. When I worked nights, I could take them to school and then go home to bed and sleep. I knew where they were and I didn't have to worry about them. I woke up in time to pick them up from school and have dinner with them before my next shift. It worked out well for my husband who was also a shift worker at the time. It was not great for our marriage, but those are the sacrifices we were willing to make for the short years our children were in primary school.

Everyone has a different story about what they're dealing with when it comes to shift work, but there are some important things to know about the supports people need when they choose shift work for the long haul.

Maya Angelou, a poet and civil rights activist said, "If you don't like something, change it; if you can't change it, change your attitude."

## The need for sleep

I know a lot of nurses who don't sleep particularly well. Many worry about their patients, their workload and the interactions of the day. Other reasons may include the addition to the family of a new baby, a sick family member or even the death of a person they loved. Sleep is important for overall health and each person needs to determine how much he or she needs to function well.

\* \* \*

Kim was not sleeping well lately. She was adjusting to her teenage daughter dating and initially the communication between them was vague. She wasn't sharing a name, age or any details of her date. It was a bit alarming for Kim that her daughter, Sam, was growing up so quickly. She lay awake at night and worried—where was Sam and what time would she be coming home? On nights when Kim was at work, she worried that she wasn't around to check in and be there to hear or see her coming in the door so that she could interpret her mood or be available for a chat. Kim wanted to let her daughter know she accepted her maturity and her ability to make good dating decisions. She also worried about that attitude coming across as giving license to promiscuity. The worry continued for a few weeks and a co-worker noticed that Kim was not herself when she was on night shift. She was being a bit short and snappy and not her usual jovial self. She put it down to lack of sleep. When Kim reflected, she realized that her worry was that Sam wasn't sharing who she was with or where she was going.

Kim decided it was time to have a heart-to-heart with Sam and share her worries. When they talked, Kim learned that her daughter was agreeable to sharing and thought her mom's lack of questioning was a sign that she didn't care. Both Kim and Sam felt better after that—this chat put them at ease and reinforced their loving relationship.

\* \* \*

When you can't show up when you want to– to be a part of family events for example– it can be distressing. It takes effort to communicate with loved ones when you can't see them as often as you would like.

We can all get by on a few hours of sleep in a pinch, but for longevity and health, doing this long-term is not sustainable. I see nurses working two and three jobs to make ends meet or to support other family members, further compromising their sleep. Then they wonder why they get sick!

**Along with diet and exercise, sleep is one of the three key pillars of health.[36] But while we often discuss food and physical fitness, sleep gets far less focus. After all, a little tiredness didn't hurt anybody, right? Wrong!**

Sleep deprivation has been shown to be just as dangerous as being intoxicated while driving. Statistics from the National Sleep Foundation refer to a study by researchers in Australia. The study showed that being awake for eighteen hours produced an impairment equal to a blood alcohol concentration (BAC) of 0.05%. If your BAC is 0.05%, that means that you have 50 milligrams of alcohol in 100 millilitres of blood. Being awake for twenty-four hours produces the equivalent of a BAC of 0.10. In Canada, 0.08 is considered legally drunk and is a criminal offence. You are three times more likely to be in a car crash if you are fatigued.[37]

A driver might not even know when he or she is fatigued, because signs of fatigue are hard to identify. Some people may also experience micro-sleep: short, involuntary moments of inattention. A micro-sleep of just four or

36    https://www.rmit.edu.au/news/all-news/2019/march/sleep-deprivation

37    https://www.nsc.org/road-safety/safety-topics/fatigued-driving

five seconds can result in a vehicle traveling the length of a football field if the driver is driving at highway speed.

The function of sleep has mystified scientists for thousands of years but modern research is providing new clues about what it does for both the mind and body.[38] Sleep serves to reenergize the body's cells, clear waste from the brain and support learning and memory. It even plays vital roles in regulating mood, appetite, and libido.

When you begin to neglect your healthy habits or hobbies, missing those feel-good parts of your day can make you vulnerable to ill health. The immune system crashes and you suffer the consequences. If you feel sluggish when working nights, especially in the early morning hours, try moving in your chair, bending forward or back or side to side. If you are able to get up and move around, that's even better. Stretching gets the blood flowing and re-energizes your system.

Donna Eden [39] has an energy exercise that involves thumping on the K27 points of the body. These points are located one inch below and lateral to your collarbone, at the top of your sternum. Thumping and breathing deeply

---

38    https://www.scientificamerican.com/article/
what-happens-in-the-brain-during-sleep1

39    Donna Eden is a pioneer in the field of energy medicine. She speaks to audiences around the world and is consulted frequently within both traditional and alternative health-care settings. Exercise taken from Donna Eden's book, *Energy Medicine*, 2008
For more information, visit www.innersource.net

stimulates your kidney meridian pathway. Try it the next time you feel drowsy. Try it before you drive home—it may prevent an accident.

Watching your diet is important, too. You may love your sugary snacks for quick bursts of energy, but unfortunately, they also make you feel drowsy a while after they are eaten and they're not the best choice for a twelve-hour shift. The same goes for coffee. Drink enough water to hydrate you and eat fruits and veggies. They may not be what you crave but you could add some pizzazz by adding a favourite dip.

**Sleep Hygiene Tips**

As your routine changes, you must change your habits to keep yourself healthy. This includes exercise. If you have a regular exercise time when you work day shift, you must also find a way to schedule an exercise time for your night shift. Don't just wait until you return to your day shift to get back on track.

I have talked about the health of our bodies and the need to support a healthy lifestyle. What can you do in your bedroom to ensure a restful sleep? Here are some ideas to consider.

Before going to bed, some people find that taking a warm bath or shower is relaxing. A shaman named Debra King once told me that adding a cup of sea salt and a cup of bicarbonate of soda to your bath water helps to take away the negative energy accumulated in your energy field during your work day.

Turning off all electronics and keeping them outside of your sleep area is helpful. The electromagnetic effects of electronic devices, specifically our cellphones, are controversial but they may have negative effects on our body. If your devices are turned off and placed outside your bedroom, that potential effect is eliminated and they cannot demand that you check messages or answer them.

Tell your friends and family when you'll be on a night shift and not to call between certain daytime hours— unless there's an emergency, of course. (For some people, you may have to define what an emergency is!) Get someone else to handle the messages or set up calls to go to voice mail or an answering machine.

Keep the room dark with blackout drapes, if possible, or blinds that block out the light. Turn clocks away from you so the light doesn't wake you when you turn over. Wearing a mask can help. Some people wear masks with aromatherapy oils such as lavender to promote calming and sleep. You'll need to find a system that works for you.

Have a fan (or something else) that creates white noise in your room. This may help you get a more restful sleep.

Addressing all of your senses helps to soothe and relax your system into sleep. Your body's circadian rhythm works best when you sleep at night. If you are working on a night shift, your body is working against the natural rhythm of light and darkness, so you need to simulate night to help you get a restful sleep.

Remember that alcohol, although initially a relaxant, will stimulate you to wake up a few hours after ingestion as its effects wear off, so your sleep may be disturbed and not restorative.

Choose comfortable sleep clothing and pay attention to your sheets, pillows and mattress, as well. A good mattress and a pillow that supports your neck and spine is worth the investment.

I went through a phase of buying a new pillow every couple of months until I found one that supported me well so that I stopped waking up with a sore neck.

## Brain Wave Patterns

The following excerpt was taken from the founder and CEO of Bulletproof, Dave Asprey. He is an American entrepreneur and author who blogs and talks on Bulletproof radio with guests invited to share from their expertise on anything from diets and supplements and ways to improve cognitive performance, heart rate variability and more. He wrote this following blog[40]: "Your brain has electricity running through it all the time. Electrical signals work with chemicals (dopamine, serotonin, oxytocin and so on) to create your experience of the world. The brain's electrical

40   Dave Asprey American entrepreneur, author and blog
https://blog.bulletproof.com/alpha-brain-waves-lower-stress

activity can be measured with an electroencephalogram (EEG). The EEG machine will show waves of electricity that travel across your brain in a regular, repeating pattern. These are brain waves, and they have a huge effect on how you think and feel. There are a few different types of brainwaves, each with different effects and can play a role in how successful you are at managing your stress.

Beta waves mediate attention and sometimes produce anxiety. Beta waves are present during our day-to-day activities of wakefulness.

Theta waves rise during drowsiness and daydreaming. They can also increase your sense of connectedness with people around you.

Delta waves increase during restorative sleep and are the deepest and slowest brain waves.

Then there are alpha waves. Alpha waves give you a feeling of deep calm, coupled with productivity, creativity and effortless focus. In this state, the body is resting between the conscious and subconscious states—this is what you experience when you are in the "flow," when you are fully immersed in an activity and lose track of time.

There is also a gamma wave pattern which is dominant when we are awake and is associated with processing information, learning, and memory."

The four states of consciousness include being awake, asleep, dreaming and during meditation. Awake, asleep, and dreaming are common to us and I will deal more with the meditative state in the next chapter.

All of these states of sleep and consciousness are necessary for optimal health of our minds, bodies and spirits.

In Dr. Martin Moore-Ede's *Working Nights Health & Safety Guide*,[41] he shares practical tips for shift workers and others who work at night.

In a nutshell, he says:

> "Your body is designed to sleep at night, making night work a challenge. Virtually all of your bodily functions have circadian rhythms and these are controlled by the biological clock in your brain. This clock, in turn, is influenced by sunlight and darkness. Understanding how your body works is a first step toward successfully coping with shift work."

*At Work*, Issue 60, April 2010: Institute for Work & Health, Toronto stated, "We live in a 24/7 world where there's work to be done from sundown to sunrise. For more than a quarter of Canada's employees, that means working shifts."[42] The key message of the article was that

---

41    https://www.amazon.ca/Working-Nights-Health-Safety-Guide/dp/0964889323 Moore-Ede, Martin. *Working Nights Health & Safety Guide.* Circadian Information. Cambridge, Mass, 1997

42    .https://www.iwh.on.ca/summaries/issue-briefing/shift-work-and-health

"...long-term night shift workers probably have an elevated risk of breast cancer, and a potentially elevated risk of colorectal cancer." In addition, "...elevated risks of gastrointestinal disorders, mental health problems (including depression) and preterm delivery during pregnancy are also found among shift workers."

It was also observed that people who work night shifts are likely to sleep less and/or have poorer sleep quality than those who work day shifts regularly.

Also, the above referenced *At Work*, Issue 60 article, stated that "Shift workers, especially those working at night, face a higher risk of workplace injury than regular day workers. Promising approaches to mitigating the adverse effects of shift work include restricting successive evening or night shifts to three shifts, limiting weekend work, moving from backward to forward shift rotation, and using a participatory approach to the design of shift schedules."

### The Heart of the Matter

The association between shift work and heart disease is not confirmed.

Isn't it interesting that heart disease is the number one cause of death in North America, and emotions are the one thing least talked about in connection to this?

The heart chakra in the centre of your chest is the home of your emotional state. When you can talk openly and safely to release your emotions, it gives you the connection and love that you need the most. Keeping secrets and staying distant and disconnected from your emotions builds a wall that keeps others out, but it also keeps your emotions trapped inside and harms your emotional well-being and physically can show up as a heart disease.

## Journaling

One way I have learned to release emotional heart pain is to write about it. Think about your hand as an extension of your heart as you write. It's a great way to heal. If you are alone and working the night shift is getting you down, try writing about it and your feelings. Let your words flow onto the page and don't edit as you go. You don't have to read your journal notes later to analyze your thoughts. The purpose is about acknowledging your feelings in that moment with acceptance and without judgment.

If you eat, exercise and sleep right but you don't look after your emotional health, you are not looking after your overall health. As the World Health Organization (WHO) states, "without mental health, there can be no true physical health."

In my experience, the number of medical incidents and deaths of patients usually occur during the night shift when there are fewer staff members to organize a resource team to support an incident if needed. Therefore, it's important that you are prepared to deal with potential stressors. Remember Murphy's Law, "Anything that can go wrong will go wrong."

It's important to know who your key emergency contacts are and how best to communicate with them, if needed. The worst time to learn a procedure is the time you have to do it under stress. It is everyone's responsibility to get properly trained. Ask for support and be safe.

## How to SHIFT:    Experiment with your routine

If you don't feel refreshed when you wake up, plan to go to bed half an hour earlier the next time and see if that makes a difference. Know the number of hours you require to feel refreshed and keep experimenting until you find the right formula. Of course, as you transition through different stages and ages, you need to re-examine your routine and adjust accordingly.

Sometimes people get stuck because a routine has worked for a long time and they get upset when it doesn't work anymore.

Try saying to yourself, "I choose to wake up rested and alert," rather than, "I'm going to be so tired and it will be hard to get through this next shift."

Say each statement a few times and ask yourself which one makes you feel better, and which makes you feel worse. Remember, your thoughts are only powerful when you attach meaning to them and they can go on to affect your mood and your behaviour.

I participated in an experiment years ago on how my thoughts could affect cooked rice. Really! I was instructed to place a small amount of cooked rice into two see through containers that had sealed lids. On one container I placed a sticky note on the lid that had the expression of a smile and on the other I placed a sticky note with the upside-down smile denoting a sad face.

I was to place both containers in the fridge. Every day, I was to open the fridge door and express happy thoughts and kind words to the "happy" container and harsh unkind words to the "sad" container. I kept this up for six months. My experiment found that the "happy" container had white rice as seen the day I put it in the fridge six months earlier. However, the "sad" container had turned the rice black beneath the lid and flecks of black throughout the container could be seen.

It made me wonder about the power of my own thoughts towards myself and how my system may be reacting to kind or unkind thoughts. It certainly brought awareness to my thoughts and to appreciate how I felt after saying positive statements versus feeling put down after the negative ones. Maybe you want to try it for yourself and see what results you get?

Another way of shifting could be to go for a walk outside in nature before you sleep, taking in the greenery and beauty to relax and rest.

Learning ways to cope and maintain your health when you are physically, mentally, socially and spiritually drained takes resources and skill. There are days when that seems impossible to do.

In the next chapter I will tell you about a compassionate approach to help you get through those difficult days.

# CHAPTER 9:
# Getting to Calm to Carry On

*What lies behind you and what lies in front of you*
*pales in comparison to what lies inside you.*

—*Ralph Waldo Emerson*

One of the most difficult experiences for a nurse to endure is the death of a patient. That's the ultimate stressor. You always remember the first death you encounter at work. I remember the death I witnessed when I was eighteen. I had been in nursing school for only three months. We had spent time in the classroom, learning theory and practicing skills before we got to experience a practicum of three months on "the wards." I was at a woman's bedside on a medical unit and a doctor was working beside me when suddenly it got very confusing. He shouted for a dressing tray and scalpel to do a "cut down." The woman had collapsed and he needed to get an intravenous line in for her medications.

I didn't know exactly what he was going to do with the scalpel, but I rushed to the clinic room to get one. In class, we had been taught that taking a dressing tray to a patient's bedside would be considered an aseptic technique and so I went about washing my hands, donning my mask and wiping down the trolley to disinfect it before I placed the dressing tray on the trolley to bring to the patient's bedside. As I was cleaning the trolley, I heard this booming voice in the doorway, "God dammit, woman, what are you doing?"

Bewildered, I jumped at his tone of voice—I didn't have a clue what he meant. I was a newbie– how did I know there was a different procedure for emergency situations? I was just doing what I had been taught! I was stunned and speechless.

The poor woman didn't make it. I hadn't formed a relationship with her and she had no family at her side and that made me feel very sad. The doctor left the bedside along with others who had arrived to assist him. I was left with the nurse who was the mentor I was assigned to that day. She wasn't looking too happy with my performance either, and together, we prepared the body for the morgue. I don't remember any family or priest visiting or being contacted before we prepped her body.

It was the first time I had seen a dead body. My only experience with death before that was attending the funeral of a class friend who had died of leukemia at the age of sixteen. It was a closed coffin service and so I had not seen his body.

The woman's skin quickly mottled and turned blue. It became cold and hardened as we worked. We washed her body and brushed her hair respectfully in silence. When she was ready and the appropriate paper work was done, we drew back the drapes surrounding us and pulled the drapes around all the beds surrounding hers so we could wheel her out of the unit unseen.

Nobody talked about her death. It was business as usual—everyone seemed so cold. How did the other nurses manage to go about their duties as though nothing had happened? I didn't ask. I was afraid I was missing something I was supposed to know and hadn't yet learned.

I went home to my apartment alone and cried. I felt inadequate, embarrassed and helpless. I knew that death is a part of life, but that day I experienced how real and raw it really was. Sometimes it's expected and we can plan the end of life with the patient and their family. But sometimes, it's sudden and shocking and the unexpected throws us off balance and makes us question our actions.

When a patient dies, the families are devastated, as expected. What a nurse can do well is to use her skill at being present to calm the tension. Words are often not needed—a compassionate touch and a look of concern to let them know that you are there for them as they go through this difficult time are often enough.

I worked for several years in long-term care and I witnessed many deaths, some peaceful and others more difficult. I've always felt honoured to be with a dying person as they left their body. Those with a faith in a higher being offer prayers and rituals to prepare the departing soul. Some faiths believe in life after death and they have their own rituals to support that soul to find its way.

As nurses, our place is not to judge, but to accept and support the wishes of the dying person as best we can. We get close to some families and patients in our care and no matter how many times we experience the death of a patient, it doesn't make it any easier. Nurses and others in the helping professions learn to tolerate the discomfort of another person's suffering and learn how to show compassion.

In my current role, I support staff when they need to take time out of their busy day to stop, get together and debrief when they have experienced something beyond what they can endure and their capacity to function has reached its limit. I support allowing staff to request time away from their responsibilities to normalize their feelings and emotions with each other.

Debriefs are controversial—are they beneficial or do they trigger attendees into more trauma? In my experience, I believe that debriefs are beneficial. I agree with Stephen Porges, PhD, who writes in his work on the Polyvagal theory, that we are hard-wired for social engagement. We can settle our nervous system by helping each other through the tough stuff– we can reconnect and feel that we are a part of the team. It strengthens relationships within the team because members are recognized for being there and doing their jobs. Helping each other to feel less isolated and alone under stress is actually a mechanism for survival. When we don't come together and talk, our nervous systems can get triggered and, consequently, our mental health may suffer.

\* \* \*

Kim was working on labour and delivery. This is usually a happy place of smiles and celebrations as new babies are born. Parents, grandparents and other family members are often milling around, waiting for the highly anticipated news of the baby's arrival—*Is baby okay? Is Mom okay?* When things go wrong in labour and delivery, they can go horribly wrong very quickly and the whole unit feels and reacts in unison to support the baby, the mom and the family, as a professional team does.

On this particular day, the vital signs of a baby—audible using the fetal monitor attached to Mom—just stopped. Kim was covering for the nurse who was in charge of Mom and baby, while the other nurse took her break. She made some adjustments to the equipment and checked on baby again and to her horror the vital signs remained absent. When the nurse heard the pager for the attending physician to report to her assigned room, she jumped up to return and attend to her patient. What followed was a well-orchestrated team effort responding to this emergency.

As the baby was full-term it was decided that the best course of action was to do an emergency Caesarean section. The father and the family were in the waiting room, not knowing what to expect. A short time passed and then the doctor went to see the family with a concerned look that alerted the family all was not well. He shared that the baby had died. Kim went to support the family—they were devastated and angry.

*What happened?!*

*Why did it happen?!*

*Whose fault is it?!*

The father and family were looking for someone or something to blame. Kim understood that their reaction was normal, but it was hard for her to deal with it anyway.

Kim was so grateful when later, her manager hit the pause button and gathered all staff involved for a break to debrief and offer some time to share their emotions about what had happened. A learning debrief was planned for later, after the investigation had pieced together the causes of the baby's death.

\* \* \*

When you are involved in upsetting situations like this, be sure to find a safe person to talk to. The stresses that go with events like this can be overwhelming. It is not a sign of weakness to ask for help–it is part of belonging to a team that cares about you and wants you to thrive, not just survive. It's also bad for your mental health to bottle things up.

I've worked in many positions on the front lines, in management, in the community, in industry and in hospitals, too, and it is compassion for self and others that gives me hope for now and for the future of healthcare.

## Self-compassion

I like the work of Kristin Neff, PhD, a self-compassion researcher, author, and Associate Professor at the University of Texas at Austin. She has defined self-compassion as having three main components:

- **Self-kindness** – "being warm towards oneself when encountering pain and personal shortcomings, rather than criticizing and hurting oneself with negative self-talk."

The experience of making a medication error comes to mind. When you know the right way to deliver the drug to the right patient, but in a moment of distraction you do it wrong, you get that awful sick feeling when you realize what you have done. Try saying something to ease the burden of your mistake. With your compassionate inner voice try saying, "Moments like this are difficult to bear; may I learn from this the best way I can."

- **Common humanity** – "recognizing that suffering and personal failure is part of the shared
  human experience."

We fear and avoid what we don't understand. When staff
are over-worked and reacting in ways that cause conflict
with co-workers, I encourage nurses to have conversations
to support each other and to decrease the stigma attached
to emotional and mental needs. Through these conversations, we discover that we are more alike than not and we
are not alone in the way we feel under stress.

- **Mindfulness** – "a non–judgmental state of mind in
  which individuals observe their thoughts and feelings as they are without trying to suppress or deny
  them, accepting them as they are."

When you slow down and pay attention to the task at
hand or the patient in front of you, you can stay present
and focused. It's a good place to be. People sense when you
are not listening to them and that your mind has drifted
to thoughts of what's next or what needs doing. The more
mindful you are, the better quality of care you can deliver
to your patients.

Dr. Neff believes that the number one reason that
people are not more self-compassionate is a belief that
self-compassion will undermine our motivation. There is
a belief that we need to be self-critical in order to motivate
ourselves to do better next time and that if we are kind to
ourselves or compassionate, we lose our motivation to act

S.H.I.F.T. Stress

in a way that is required. She goes on to say, "For many years, self-esteem was seen to be the key to psychological health. However, research psychologists have identified several downsides to the endless pursuit of self-esteem such as ego-defensiveness, constant social comparisons and instability of self-worth. Research suggests that self-compassion is a healthier way of relating to oneself, offering all the benefits of self-esteem without its downsides.

"Self-compassion involves treating ourselves kindly, like we would a good friend we care about.

**"Rather than continually judging and evaluating ourselves, self-compassion involves generating kindness toward ourselves as imperfect humans, and learning to be present with the inevitable struggles of life with greater ease.**

"It motivates us to make needed changes in our lives, not because we're worthless or inadequate, but because we care about ourselves and want to lessen our suffering."

According to Dr. Neff, there has been an explosion of research into self-compassion over the past decade and the studies strongly link self-compassion to feelings of well-being, less anxiety and depression and more life satisfaction. When we are more present to ourselves as compassionate human beings, we can also show up for others through our connectedness, curiosity and gratitude.

When we embrace our own suffering with care and kindness, it soothes our negative states and helps to integrate the parts of us that we have been denying which helps to take us to a more positive place.

**Take a self-compassion break**

Another way to add a moment of relaxation into your busy day is by doing a "self-compassion break" exercise by Dr. Neff.[43] Practice putting your hand on different parts of your body, for example your chin, chest, abdomen, elbow or even holding on to a finger. Take several breaths while touching this body part and see if you notice a shift in your tension. Once you find a spot that helps relax you then this will become an anchor for your mind and body to associate a way to release your tension. You can then think of a situation that is causing you stress or some difficulty that you are dealing with in your life.

Say to yourself, "This is stress" (the mindful part of being self-compassionate).

Then you can say to yourself, "Other people feel this way, too" (which is the common humanity part of self-compassion). And lastly, you may say to yourself, "May I learn to accept myself as I am" (this is the self-kindness part of self-compassion). You can add any statement that you prefer, whatever your intention is. This exercise evokes the three aspects of self-compassion when you need it most.

---

43   https://self-compassion.org/exercise-2-self-compassion-break/

## Compassion fatigue and the cost of caring

All health care providers are at risk of Compassion Fatigue. As it turns out, when you are good at doing the work you do—giving to others in your care—it can take a toll on your own health. It could be considered an occupational hazard. To date, there are no agreed upon terms to describe this condition, so I am referring to the training material I received from the "Compassion Fatigue: Train the Trainer Workbook" 2017, by Françoise Mathieu, the founder of the TEND Academy[44] that I attended in 2018.

> **Compassion or caregiver fatigue** (CF) manifests as an erosion of our compassion and refers to the marked emotional and physical wearing down that takes place when health care providers are unable to refuel themselves.
>
> **Vicarious Trauma (VT) or Secondary Trauma Stress (STS)** have been used to describe the profound affect that workers experience in their world view when they work with clients who have experienced trauma. VT is the repeated exposure to difficult stories, events or witnessing a horrific scene. Health care providers may find it difficult to rid themselves of the experience and become intensely preoccupied with it. This experience may alter their view of the world they live in. For example, if you

---

44    Further information at www.tendacademy.ca

witness a plane crash, it may no longer feel safe for you to travel on a plane. Both CF and VT/STS are experienced by the helping professions only.

**Burnout** is a physical and emotional exhaustion resulting in the depleted ability to cope with work demands. This can result in low job satisfaction, feelings of low control and high stress.

This condition can be experienced by any worker in a helping and non-helping profession.

**Moral Distress** results from inconsistencies between your personal beliefs and the requirements of your job, which can cause internal and ethical conflict. For example, legislation was passed in the Supreme Court of Canada in June 2016 allowing physician-assisted suicides. This goes against the beliefs of many doctors and nurses and can cause great distress when they are asked to take part in this type of process.

### An ABC approach to compassion fatigue

I use the ABC approach with staff to educate and validate their experience of compassion fatigue. The concept of ABC - Awareness, Balance and Connection was originally developed by Saakvitne & Pearlman in their 1996 book

"Transforming the Pain." The following are highlights from the handout.[45]

## Awareness (Self-awareness)

Self-awareness allows you to notice your own early warning signs of distress.

- Physical (for example: headaches, muscular tension, upset stomach)
- Behavioural (for example: anger and irritability)
- Spiritual and emotional (one example: a lack of meaning or purpose)
- Psychological (for example: distancing, worry, guilt and shame)

There are many symptoms that we as health care providers can identify with. Different people will react differently and may experience some, but not necessarily all, of these symptoms. Often those who work closely with you will recognize your symptoms before you do. Conversely, you may notice changes in others before they are aware of them themselves.

Once you are aware of your own symptoms, then you have a choice to ignore them and carry on or pay attention

---

45    Saakvitne, K. & Pearlman, L. (1996). Transforming the Pain: A Workbook on Vicarious Traumatization for Helping Professionals who Work with Traumatized Clients. New York, New York: W.W. Norton and Company.

to your needs and address them. What defense will you create for yourself?

* * *

What strategies can Kim use when she has had enough?

When Kim feels upset and needs some space to pull herself together, she was taught to use statements such as: "When I feel angry, I need to ask for a break so I can go for a walk off the unit" or "When I get nervous, I need to laugh."

* * *

Breaking the silence on our own mental health struggles takes courage. Communicating our needs to others is a step towards creating a safe place to work with compassion and non-judgment, which in turn will help build supportive, caring and, ultimately, stronger teams for our patients and ourselves.

### Balance

This doesn't mean that you have to get everything accomplished in every twenty-four period in order to have a balance in your work and home life. I'm suggesting that over the course of a week or so you could arrange to have a more give-and-take approach to work demands, home commitments and lifestyle choices. This could also include knowing what you enjoy doing that can help you to recharge when you are stressed. Could this take the pressure off you for having these unrealistic expectations?

I suggest taking breaks, which includes the biggest break of all– as in making sure that you take your vacation time. I know that isn't always possible when you need it, but finding some time every day, to unplug, even if for five minutes, to focus on your own self-care, is so important for your mental health.

If massage is included in your benefits, then by all means, maximize your use of it. Massages help to relax and re-energize you and it's great for everyone including singles, widows or widowers—anyone not in intimate relation-ships—to get the benefits of relaxation with safe touch.

Also, consider the practice of meditation which has been practiced for thousands of years. Originally, it was meant to help deepen understanding of the sacred and mystical forces of life. These days, meditation is commonly used for relaxation and stress reduction.[46] Many studies have shown the benefits of meditation including being able to clear away the information overload that builds up every day which may be contributing to your stress. Meditation can improve attention and concentration, enhance self-awareness and generate kindness. There are even scientific studies that look at how meditation may slow down the aging process. The excerpt below is taken from the peer

---

46   https://www.mayoclinic.org/tests-procedures/meditation/in-depth/meditation/art-20045858

reviewed article which was published in the Annals of the New York Academy of Science (2009) and is entitled "Can meditation slow the rate of cellular aging?"[47]:

*"Understanding the malleable determinants of cellular aging is critical to understanding human longevity. Telomeres may provide a pathway for exploring this question. Telomeres are the protective caps at the ends of chromosomes. The length of telomeres offers insight into mitotic cell and possibly organismal longevity. Telomere length has now been linked to chronic stress exposure and depression. This raises the question of how might cellular aging be modulated by psychological functioning.*

*We consider two psychological processes or states that are in opposition to one another--threat cognition and mindfulness--and their effects on cellular aging. Psychological stress cognitions, particularly appraisals of threat and ruminative thoughts, can lead to prolonged states of reactivity. In contrast, mindfulness meditation techniques appear to shift cognitive appraisals from threat to challenge, decrease ruminative thought, and*

---

47    E. Epil, PhD; J. Daubenmier, Phd; J.T. Moskowitz, Phd; S. Folkman, PhD; E. Blackburn, Phd: Ann N Y Acad Sci. 2009 Aug; 1172: 34-53

*reduce stress arousal. Mindfulness may also directly increase positive arousal states."*

Here's a list of other options:

- Get a good night's sleep
- Develop a buddy system to have someone to debrief with
- Step away when you need to
- Schedule your fitness
- Schedule your relaxation
- Practice coherent breathing
- Journal
- Laugh
- Make a mental list of things you are grateful for at the beginning and end of each shift
- Seek social supports at work
- Read something that relaxes you or stimulates your personal growth
- Seek a mentor to support how you may balance your workload and re-prioritize as the day goes along
- Limit listening to the details of difficult stories or also any gossip–stop the drama
- Improve your own work/life integration in a way that works for you

- Develop resiliency through the practice of habits that sustain you and engage you
- Get coaching or counselling to support yourself
- But most important, be self-compassionate!

**Self-care is not optional for health care workers; it is required to maintain a healthy mind, body and spirit to cope with the demands of each day.**

Caregivers who are self-compassionate have increased satisfaction and less burnout–it's a powerful protective factor.

Self-care is self-full, not selfish. Many people may perceive some of these self-care practices as selfish, but they are not. In fact, if you participate in self-care, you are more likely to be a better giver to others and a more effective health care provider.

As part of my training in compassion fatigue I learned a way to connect to myself and recognize the signals that I needed self-care. The following quote offers you a way to do this too.

"We need to gain a better understanding of our own warning signs along the continuum of compassion fatigue. Using traffic lights as an analogy, the green zone is where you are when you are at your very best. The yellow zone is where most of us live most of the time. We have warning signs emerging but we often ignore them. The red zone is the danger zone."[48] Being aware of your early warning signs, can you identify when you shift from a green light to a yellow?

When I ask people what "turns their green light to yellow," and what is happening to create this change, I often hear things like additional admissions or discharges (more work/paperwork), working short-staffed (co-workers called in sick) and emergency codes requiring response. These are hospital scenarios and I'm sure that in other settings, you have similar situations that can cause you to go from a calm green state to an increasingly stressful one—that can alert you that you are entering into the yellow caution zone.

Then I ask them what helps bring them back from a yellow light to a green. They often find this difficult to articulate. Some feel they are stuck at yellow for the remainder of the shift. Some come into work on green and it doesn't take much to push them to yellow. If they stay in the yellow zone for a prolonged period and are not aware of their early warning signs and do not put effort into a recovery plan to get back into the green zone, it's just a matter of time before they escalate into the red zone. This could show up, for example, as anger and conflict. This may cause a worker to break down and cry and find reasons to stop work and go home. We often recognize the red light in these people. These co-workers may be at

---

48    Mathieu, Françoise. The Compassion Fatigue Workbook. Routledge Taylor & Francis Group 2012, pg 48

work physically, but not mindfully present, at work—this is called presenteeism. Others in this red zone represent a percentage of workers who are off sick and hopefully receiving treatment and recovering.

Those able to make their own shift back to green say that some of the things that help them are taking a break, eating a snack, giving and receiving hugs, participating in debriefs and praying.

We talk about balance and what they could include in their daily routine to promote returning to green. I encourage health care professionals to check their awareness of their work environments to see what they can do to support each other to return to the calm of a green light.

### Connection

C stands for connection. It's important to be able to reach out for support and connect with the resources you have available to you in your workplace.

C also stands for commitment—what can you do in the next week, month or year to support your self-care plan?

## Self-Care for Health Care Workers

Self-care is taking responsibility for yourself.
Self-care is creating boundaries that enhance your well-being.

Self-care is saying "yes" to things/people that create a sense of joy and a feeling of expanded energy inside you.

Self-care is saying "no" to things/people that make your energy and mood contract, and don't feel good inside you.

Self-care is creating your own "first aid kit" and using it when needed.

Self-care is creating moments to fill yourself up before you can give again.

Self-care is learning to give to yourself first.

Self-care is not self-absorption or being narcissistic; it is loving-kindness.

Self-care is being aware of your limitations and accepting those limitations.

Self-care is knowing that suffering is part of being human.

Self-care is knowing that growth and change is a choice.

Self-care is asking for help when it's needed.

Self-care is being safe and trusting your own intuition.

Self-care is letting go of the day and allowing time for rest and play.

Self-care is not a choice; it is required for your optimal health.

Self-care can prevent burnout, compassion fatigue and vicarious trauma.

Self-care is self-compassion.

Self-care is a commitment to yourself.

Self-care because nobody else can.

I created these statements to provide some ideas of what self-care could mean for individuals. I invite you to read the statements and pick one or two that you find relatable and can use as a mantra to remind yourself why your self-care practice is important to you. It's also a good idea to share your self-care goal with a buddy to help increase the likelihood that you commit to the practice of your self-care goal and achieve it. Below is an example of how you could set up a commitment statement:

Today on this date: _____, I commit
to my self-care by doing (one of the statements, above):

_____

_____

I'm sharing this with my buddy to support
me (name)_____

_____

_____

Signature:

## How to SHIFT: Be mindful in your day

Decide which of the statements above resonate with you
and add them to your tool box. We'll talk more about how
to put this all together in the next chapter.

Mindfulness is about slowing down the mind and
paying attention to your thoughts with acceptance and
non-judgment. On a busy day, we are not thinking about
slowing our minds or being mindful, we are focused on
accomplishing what we need to do. Our training takes over
and carries us through the tasks at hand.

Here's how to shift by being mindful during your
work day: In the few seconds or minutes between tasks
or between patients, notice your thoughts, feelings and
sensations. For example, while you are washing your hands,
in those twenty seconds, notice your breathing and say a

kind word to yourself. Or, as you walk between patient rooms, pay attention to the way you are walking, first your right leg and foot and then your left as you connect to the floor with each step—your mindful walk can bring you back to the present moment.

When you are present to what is happening in this moment, it interrupts any negative cycle you may have going on in your mind. You cannot keep other thoughts in your mind when you are in the present moment. The more you are present in your day, the more it builds a capacity of tolerance to expand those moments, helping you lead a happier, healthier life.

It would be remiss of me not to mention the work of Jon Kabat-Zinn, PhD, the founder of the mindfulness-based stress reduction program that is based on sound scientific research and offered around the world. His work is well documented in his book titled Full Catastrophe Living. It offers ways to live a life to support health and happiness. [49]

The following exercise draws on a guided meditation by researcher Emma Seppala, Science Director of Stanford University's Center for Compassion and Altruism Research and Education.

Using a mantra to support yourself, when you have an unkind thought towards yourself or others, helps to soften your response and increases your compassion

---

49    Kabat-Zinn, Jon, PhD *Full Catastrophe Living: Using the Wisdom of Your Body and Mind to Face Stress, Pain, and Illness.* Bantam Dell ,Delta trade paperback reissue, January 2005

toward yourself and others, too. [50] The original name of this practice is metta bhavana, which comes from the Pali language, native to the Indian subcontinent. Metta means 'love' (in a non-romantic sense), friendliness, or kindness: hence 'loving-kindness' for short. It is an emotion, something you feel in your heart. Bhavana means development or cultivation. [51]

There are many variations and this is just one. You can sit in a comfortable position with an erect back focusing on being aware. As you say silently to yourself some of the following phrases reflect and notice how you receive them in your heart.

The Loving Kindness Metta meditation goes like this:

May I be safe

May I be healthy

May I be at peace

May I accept whatever comes

May I have the courage to face my fears

May I be forgiving

May I be happy

May I live with ease

---

50   https://ggia.berkeley.edu/practice/loving_kindness_meditation
Emma Seppala, PhD is also the author of *The Happiness Track* (HarperOne

51   https://thebuddhistcentre.com/text/loving-kindness-meditation

Pick two or three statements and carry them with you until you've memorized them. Practice and repeat.

You can also offer this to others in your family, neighbours or co-workers you see in distress by saying, in your mind:

> May you be safe
>
> May you be healthy
>
> May you be at peace

We can also offer this to the larger community we live in and even globally:

> May we be safe
>
> May we be healthy
>
> May we be at peace

"Getting calm to carry on" means finding ways to de-escalate tension, regulate your emotions and support yourself using self-compassion.

We are all in this together. In being a part of the human race, we share the suffering of others, so it makes sense to ask: *Why would I want to add to the suffering of the world with my unkind thoughts or words?*

# CHAPTER 10:
# Arranging your tools to help you cope

*If there is light in the heart, there will be beauty in the person.*
*If there is beauty in the person, there will be harmony in*
*the house.*
*If there is harmony in the house, there will be order in*
*the nation.*
*If there is order in the nation, there will be peace in the world.*

*—Chinese Proverb*

We want beauty, harmony, order and peace in our lives. My intention for you is to find new practices to shift your sense of self and to experience more harmony in your life.

I didn't have the tools I needed when I experienced burnout. In my early thirties, with a young family, shift work and school and with no family supports, I didn't know that I needed better tools to cope with life. I just expected myself to do what was needed for myself and my family. There was certainly no time for social outlets.

But we are social beings who need connection. The moments of connection and life with others are the moments that sustain and support our growth and vitality. Without them, we become disconnected, lonely and isolated.

Looking back at my workplace at the time I was raising my children, I remember that I was able to share my stories and listen to the stories of my co-workers, along with the other young moms and nurses. Although I wasn't aware of it at the time, it gave me strength to cope. Later, when I left that workplace, it became very evident that something was missing.

When you stop doing the things that sustain you, such as connecting with friends, or going for a walk or to the gym, because other things have taken priority over your time, you become distracted from your social connections and over time, you will find that your ability to cope is reduced, as I learned the hard way.

I had to learn that needing "me time" to re-energize was not selfish; self-care was necessary so that I could do the everyday things that were expected from my job and my family and the things I wanted to do.

As I stepped back, I recognized that my job gave me great satisfaction and enjoyment but my marriage relationship did not. I decided it was time to face my fears and talk about my concerns for the future. It was a difficult time—separating—but one I don't regret. I wanted to be a good role model for my then four teenage daughters and that meant that staying in an unhealthy relationship was not okay.

Over time, that experience went from vulnerability to a strength for me. I'm now able to see the gift of that experience and use it as I counsel young moms and nurses who are having difficulty in their relationships. I want to make a difference with the coping tools I have learned and pass these on to help other people's relationships survive their challenges. If I am able to help others to reach out and not suffer alone, then I will have achieved my goal in writing this book.

I didn't know what resources were available nor was I offered any help when I most needed it. I didn't look like I needed any help on the outside so why would anybody offer it? And I didn't know how to ask. I don't know if it would have made a difference to the outcome of my marriage, but I do know that I am not alone in the struggle to understand relationships. It takes an interest and a caring, loving presence to listen with compassion and empathy. All relationships are like a mirror in which we see ourselves more clearly if we are willing to be curious and willing to grow.

Have you noticed in your own life that the time you experienced the most adversity was also the time you experienced the most growth?

I look at challenging times differently now—as an opportunity to reflect and grow. These are times to use my tools to recover and get back on my feet.

If you are reading this book because you are struggling with stress in your life and you are looking for solutions, I am happy to tell you that there are tremendous resources available and you don't have to do it without support.

## Adding to your "toolbox"

I want you to take the tools from this book and add your own to create a toolbox that works for you. If you're like me in needing order, consider following the nursing assessment process: assess your needs, plan how you will use and practice with your new tools and then evaluate how well each one works for you. Remember that you can change the tools and rearrange them as the years go by to suit your emotional needs.

Here is a brief review of the tools we have learned in each chapter:

| | |
|---|---|
| **Chapter 2** | Take a stress test to increase your awareness of your stress and how it is affecting your life |
| | Shift using the coherent breathing technique |
| | Name your physical symptoms when you notice that you aren't feeling right and stretch or breathe into the tension |
| | Use compassionate self-talk to soothe the stress you feel in that moment |
| **Chapter 3** | Consider that your beliefs could be contributing to your stress and remind yourself of the Serenity Prayer |
| | Try to name a cognitive distortion you may be carrying and reframe your self-talk when your automatic negative thoughts (ANTs) come up |

**Chapter 4**    Try courageous conversations to find your voice when you are under stress
Work on your communication style—can you reduce the stress and conflict around you?
Consider chakra meditations to connect and balance your inner body/energy field
Try journaling to help release stress that's become stuck
Do a zip-up exercise to protect your energy

**Chapter 5**    Do a body scan to find out where you are holding tension and figure out what triggered you to react
Use the SHIFT technique to take you from a reaction to a response
Try the HALT technique to help avoid trigger states
Use the Emotional Freedom Technique (EFT) to reduce stress

**Chapter 6**    Practice being assertive and work on maintaining healthy boundaries
Learn your attachment style; choose relationships that support your style
Learn your "window of tolerance" and try to understand what kinds of things trigger you
Learn what to do when you feel triggered

**Chapter 7**    Identify your sub-personalities– explore these sub-personalities and consider how understanding these can help you support yourself when under stress

**Chapter 8**    Work on learning ways to cope with the stress of shift work, especially if you have to work night shifts
Examine your sleep hygiene and make changes that will improve the quality of your rest

**Chapter 9**    Practice being calm under tension
Use self-compassion to be kind towards yourself when challenges show up. Try the self-compassion exercise or loving kindness meditation.
Try meditation to help resolve your stress and calm your mind; choose or make up a self-care statement

Remember: Use your nursing process on yourself: assess, plan, implement and evaluate.

## How to SHIFT : *Using some of these tools together*

*Example*

Create your plan for using the tools and form new habits provided throughout this book to practice your self-care. Start by writing each of the tools you would like to use under the heading that seems most appropriate by taking a piece of paper and dividing it into three columns. The three columns represent your work day. Label them "BEFORE," "DURING" and "AFTER."

For example, under "BEFORE," you could:
- write an intention for your day
- say an affirmation such as "May I be safe, may I be healthy, may I be at peace," or
- say these words while doing the energy zip-up exercise
- Under "DURING," when stressors arise through your work day, you could write:
- body scan to relax
- breathe and stretch
- debrief after an event
- hug, smile, laugh and be compassionate- these are all good choices, too.

In the "AFTER" column, you could write "EFT" and tap on any stressors that you experienced. You could also add tools like:
- spend time with friends

- talk on the phone
- read a good book
- watch a movie
- do a five-minute meditation
- cook
- garden
- walk
- go to the gym

Carry the paper with you and put it in a place that will remind you how important your self-care is to your day and all its benefits—not only for you but also for all the people in your life.

**Review your self-care plan at the beginning or the end of each year (or as often as you feel is necessary) or add a review on your birthday to celebrate how important you are to yourself.**

In your review, ask yourself these questions:

What tools are working?

What needs tweaking?

Do any of the tools need to be replaced?

# CHAPTER 11:
# A Plug for Therapy

*Wounding and healing are not opposites. They're part
of the same thing. It is our wounds that enable us to
be compassionate with the wounds of others.*

*–Rachel Naomi Remen*

Working as a nurse and looking for resources to help others,
I didn't imagine that one day, I would be here sharing parts
of my story with you through a book. I didn't learn anything about self-care in my training to be a nurse or in my
speciality as an Occupational Health Nurse. It was through
my education to become a psychotherapist I learned the
importance of self-care.

A mentor of mine shared a story of a nine-year-old boy
who was struggling after the break-up of his parents. It
was hard for him to see the sunshine or to experience his
own light of being a fun-loving little boy until one day he

told my mentor, "Oh, I get it now. I just have to tap away the clouds and the sun will be there."

Our true self– our best self– is always there, hidden by the experiences that have clouded the way we see ourselves and our potential for life.

As a therapist I feel privileged to be a part of other people's stories. As I have worked on my own healing, I recognize that I'm still growing and learning and that we are all "works in progress". As I have come to understand and accept this, it means that there is always opportunity for growth and change until the day I die.

That's my plug for therapy. Digging where you don't want to go is not for the faint of heart but as the scholar and psychiatrist Carl Jung said (and I'm paraphrasing), "You will be more beautiful, authentic and empowered on the other side."

Everyone experiences stress at different points in their life—both good and bad. Stress can appear in response to a wedding, a move to a new home, starting a new job, giving birth, raising children and other family events. Stress can also arise as the result of the death of a loved one or the end of a marriage or to the death of a co-worker. When stress, and the symptoms associated with stress, begin to interfere with your normal functioning, it may be time to seek professional help. See your family physician and seek a therapist.

Let's support the early detection of compassion fatigue, burnout, vicarious trauma and post-traumatic stress disorder (PTSD).

Remember that you are human, too, and you have emotions and feelings that can be overwhelming, especially with the work you do as a health care professional.

I applaud all health care providers in their efforts to perform their work. I'll say it again—if you get to a point in your career that it all becomes too much to handle alone, that's okay. You are not alone. It is not okay to stay alone with these feelings. Please reach out and ask for help. There is plenty of it around but you need to invite the support. No one can read your mind and no one can do the work for you. Just as you give care for others, you sometimes have to give it back to yourself, too. Remember that good feeling you get when you help others? Allow others to help you when you need it and allow them to feel that same reward.

As I was gathering inspirational ideas for this book, I lost an afternoon on Instagram one day. I saw a photo of what looked like a graduating class of nurses. They were sitting in rows and each was holding a sign. Collectively, the signs expressed what nursing meant to them: *I save lives. I provide comfort in death. I care. Your wellbeing is my reward. I am your advocate. Nursing is my skill, but caring is my profession.* This is posted on simplenursing.com.

It is my hope that the optimism shared by these new nurses carries them through their career and that each and every one of them might develop tools to handle life's stressors as they present themselves, and thereby be able to continue to follow their positive affirmations for the remainder of their working lives.

I offer you one last tool—an old Hawaiian prayer called the "Ho'oponopo prayer":

I'm sorry

Please forgive me

Thank-you

I love you

Use this prayer when you have past hurts with somebody but you are not able to make a personal visit for various reasons, including when the person is deceased. It can bring you comfort by expressing your need for forgiveness in an otherwise hopeless situation. To get relief, repeat it as often as you need.

Remember mental health affects people of all ages, all levels of education, income levels and culture. Are you ready to SHIFT?

## How to SHIFT:      Eight steps to Self-Care

Shift your stress by knowing who in your community can offer support and resources.

Use these eight steps to help you get through your next stressful event utilizing my acronym SELF-CARE:

**S**tress test to increase awareness

**E**xamine your beliefs; ask where your stress comes from

**L**earn to engage in courageous conversations under stress

**F**ocus on using SHIFT to get from a stress reaction to a response

**C**ompassion toward yourself while under stress

**A**ccept that stress is part of the job and an opportunity to stretch and grow

**R**e-connect to mind, body and spirit to fuel your personal needs and support your purpose

**E**ngage in activities, on your own and with others, that feel good and bring out your best self

I hope that I have given you enough reasons to reach out and ask for help when you need it. I have shared the tools that work for me and my clients. Of course, there are many more resources available and new resources are being created all the time, so I hope that I have whetted your appetite to go out and look for them. Don't just accept the status quo, "It is what it is." If you get stuck, please look for help. Change is possible when you want to shift a perspective, shift your stress and change the way you think about yourself and the work you do. You will be so much better when you get to the other side!

Marcus Aurelius, a philosopher and Roman emperor, wrote this between 121AD-180AD. His words remain current and timeless for today:

**You have unlimited power over your mind, not outside events. Realize this, and you will find strength.**
*—Marcus Aurelius*

# APPENDIX A

List of sub-personalities (with permission from Transformational Arts College of Spiritual and Holistic Training)

| Sub-personality | Positive function | Negative function |
| --- | --- | --- |
| Addict | Can take pleasure and thrives with connection or attachment to something | Illusion can be difficult to disconnect and becomes self-destructive |
| Approval Seeker | Social/congenial and flexible | Not in touch with self and creates chaos |
| Caretaker | Nurturing/caring/sees wounds in others | Neglects self, creates victims |
| Chronic Crier | Expresses sadness and is trusting | Manipulative, and has no self-control |
| Comedian | Light-hearted and likeable in social situations | Can be insensitive, and not taking life seriously |
| Controller | Organized and detail oriented | Suffocates others and can create chaos and disappointment |
| Inner critic | Awareness of danger, reality check | Disabling messages and shaming |
| Fixer/Rescuer | Helpful and considerate towards others | Disempowering and neglects own pain |
| Judge | Observant and decisive | Judgmental and intolerant |

| | | |
|---|---|---|
| **Lost child** | Independent and adaptable to all situations | Lonely, disconnected, and isolated |
| **Martyr** | Dedicated | Controlling and has no boundaries. |
| **Over-Achiever** | Strives for excellence and doesn't give up easily | Easily burns out and often has high demands |
| **People pleaser** | Diplomatic and finds peaceful solution | Sells out true self and avoids conflict at all cost |
| **Perfectionist** | Responsible and gives his/her best | Rigid and creates victims or conflict |
| **Pillar of Strength/Tower** | Self-sufficient, supportive, and strong | Feels alienated/lonely and can get bitter and resentful |
| **Rebel** | Fighting for a cause and sensitive | No clear direction and angry |
| **Spiritualist** | Has faith and trust, positive and in touch with God | Spiritual bypass, and cut off from human side |
| **Teacher** | Shares information, is logical and clear thinking | Rigid, theoretical, and judgmental |
| **Victim** | In touch with feelings. Sensitive to other's pain | Manipulative, and hands over power to others |

# APPENDIX B[52]

# TAPPING POINTS

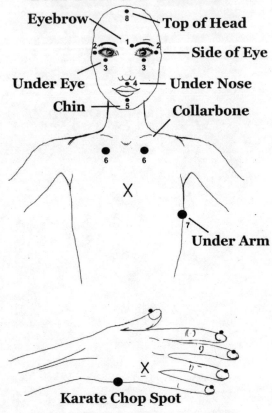

Stress relief point: Put hand over x on chest & tap x with fingertips on other hand at the same time.

# APPENDIX C

**Somatic Attachment Trainings and DARe Workshops
Know Your Adult Attachment Style Mini-Questionnaire**
© With permission from Diane Poole Heller, Ph.D. 743
Club Circle Louisville, CO 80027
www.dianepooleheller.com

Instructions:

When completing this questionnaire, please focus on one significant relationship—ideally a current or past partner, as the focus here is on adult relationships. This does not *necessarily* need to be a romantic relationship but *must* be the individual with whom you feel the most connection. Who is your primary "go to" person if you're sick, in trouble, want to celebrate, call with news, etc.

This questionnaire is designed to be an interactive learning tool. Please highlight, circle, or comment on any statements that are particularly relevant to you or that you'd like to revisit for exploration at a later time.

When responding, consider how strongly you identify with each statement. Using the scale below, respond in the space provided.

# S.H.I.F.T. Stress

| | | Disagree | Sometimes Agree | Mostly Agree | Strongly Agree |
|---|---|---|---|---|---|
| **Secure** | | **0** | **1** | **2** | **3** |
| 1 | I feel relaxed with my partner most of the time. | | | | |
| 2 | I find it easy to flow between being close and connected with my partner to being on my own. | | | | |
| 3 | If my partner and I hit a glitch, it is relatively easy for me to apologize, brainstorm a win-win solution, or repair the mis-attunement or disharmony. | | | | |
| 4 | People are essentially good at heart. | | | | |
| 5 | It is a priority to keep agreements with my partner. | | | | |
| 6 | I attempt to discover and meet the needs of my partner whenever possible, and I feel comfortable expressing my own needs. | | | | |
| 7 | I actively protect my partner from others and from harm, and attempt to maintain safety in our relationship. | | | | |
| 8 | I look at my partner with kindness and caring and look forward to our time together. | | | | |
| 9 | I am comfortable being affectionate with my partner. | | | | |
| 10 | I can keep secrets, protect my partner's privacy, and respect boundaries. | | | | |
| | Section Total | | | | |

## Avoidant

| | Disagree | Sometimes Agree | Mostly Agree | Strongly Agree |
|---|---|---|---|---|
| | **0** | **1** | **2** | **3** |
| 1 When my partner arrives home or approaches me, I feel inexplicably stressed—especially when he or she wants to connect. | | | | |
| 2 I find myself minimizing the importance of close relationships in my life. | | | | |
| 3 I insist on self-reliance; I have difficulty reaching out when I need help, and I do many of life's tasks or my hobbies, alone. | | | | |
| 4 I sometimes feel superior in not needing others and wish others were more self-sufficient. | | | | |
| 5 I feel like my partner is always there but would often prefer to have my own space unless I invite the connection. | | | | |
| 6 Sometimes I prefer casual sex instead of a committed relationship. | | | | |
| 7 I usually prefer relationships with things or animals instead of people. | | | | |
| 8 I often find eye contact uncomfortable and particularly difficult to maintain. | | | | |
| 9 It is easier for me to think things through than to express myself emotionally. | | | | |
| 10 When I lose a relationship, at first, I might experience separation elation and then become depressed. | | | | |
| Section Total | | | | |

| | Disagree | Sometimes Agree | Mostly Agree | Strongly Agree |
|---|---|---|---|---|
| **Anxious/Ambivalent** | **0** | **1** | **2** | **3** |
| 1. I am always yearning for something or someone that I feel I cannot have and rarely feeling satisfied. | | | | |
| 2. Sometimes, I over-function, over-adapt, over-accommodate others, or over-apologize for things I did not do, in an attempt to stabilize the connection. | | | | |
| 3. Over-focusing on others, I tend to lose myself in relationships. | | | | |
| 4. It is difficult for me to say NO or to set realistic boundaries. | | | | |
| 5. I chronically second-guess myself and sometimes wish I had said something differently. | | | | |
| 6. When I give more than I get, I often resent this and harbour a grudge. It is often difficult to receive love from my partner when they express it. | | | | |
| 7. It is difficult for me to be alone. If alone, I feel stressed, abandoned, hurt, and/or angry. | | | | |
| 8. At the same time as I feel a deep wish to be close with my partner, I also have a paralyzing fear of losing the relationship. | | | | |
| 9. I want to be close with my partner but feel angry at my partner at the same time. After anxiously awaiting my partner's arrival, I end up picking fights. | | | | |
| 10. I often tend to "merge" or lose myself in my partner and feel what they feel, or want what they want. | | | | |
| Section Total | | | | |

| Disorganized | Disagree | Sometimes Agree | Mostly Agree | Strongly Agree |
|---|:---:|:---:|:---:|:---:|
| | **0** | **1** | **2** | **3** |
| 1. When I reach a certain level of intimacy with my partner, I sometimes experience inexplicable fear. | | | | |
| 2. When presented with problems, I often feel stumped and feel they are irresolvable. | | | | |
| 3. I have an exaggerated startle response when others approach me unexpectedly. | | | | |
| 4. My partner often comments or complains that I am controlling. | | | | |
| 5. I often expect the worst to happen in my relationship. | | | | |
| 6. Protection often feels out of reach. I struggle to feel safe with my partner. | | | | |
| 7. I have a hard time remembering and discussing the feelings related to my past attachment situations. I disconnect, dissociate, or get confused. | | | | |
| 8. Stuck in approach-avoidance patterns with my partner, I want closeness but am also afraid of the one I desire to be close with. | | | | |

|   | | | |
|---|---|---|---|
| 9 | My instinctive, active self-protective responses are often unavailable when possible danger is present—leaving me feeling immobilized, disconnected, or "gone." | | | |
| 10 | Because I am easily confused or disoriented, especially when stressed, it is important for my partner to keep arrangements simple and clear. | | | |
| | Section Total | | | |

## Scoring:

For each section, add up your responses and record your total number. The section with the highest number will likely correspond to your unique attachment style. You may discover a dominant style or a mix of styles.

This questionnaire is not meant to be a label or diagnosis. It is only intended to indicate tendencies and prompt more useful, precise personal exploration.

# APPENDIX D

Further Reading

Amen, Daniel G. Dr. *Change your Brain, Change your Life*. Three Rivers Press. New York, NY, 1998

Anodea, Judith, PhD *Charge and the Energy Body: The Vital Key to Healing Your Life, Your Chakras and Your Relationships.* Hay House, Inc. 2018

Beck, Judith S. PhD *Cognitive Therapy: Basics and Beyond.* The Guilford Press. New York, 1995

Brown, Brene, PhD *The Gifts of Imperfection: Let Go of Who You Think You're Supposed to Be and Embrace Who You Are.* Hazelden Centre City, Minnesota, 2010

Eden, Donna, with David Feinstein, PhD *Energy Medicine: Balancing your Body's Energies for Optimal Health, Joy and Vitality.* Penguin Group. New York, NY, 1998

Greenberger, Dennis, PhD and Christine A. Padesky, PhD *Mind over Mood.* The Guilford Press. New York, 1995

Hanson, Rick, PhD *Hardwiring Happiness: The New Brain Science of Contentment, Calm and Confidence.* Penguin Random House, 2013

Johnson, Sue, PhD *Hold me Tight: Seven Conversations for a Lifetime of Love.* Little Brown Spark. New York, NY, 2008

Kabat-Zinn, Jon, PhD *Full Catastrophe Living: Using the Wisdom of Your Body and Mind to Face Stress, Pain, and Illness.* Bantam Dell Delta trade paperback reissue, January 2005

Levine, Peter, PhD A. *In an Unspoken Voice: How the Body Releases Trauma and Restores Goodness.* North Atlantic Books. Berkeley, California, 2010

Levine, Peter, PhD A. *Waking the Tiger: Healing Trauma.* North Atlantic Books. Berkeley, California, 1997

Mate, Gabor, Dr. *When the Body Says No: The Cost of Hidden Stress.* Random House. Canada, 2012

Moore-Ede, Martin Dr. *Working Nights: Health & Safety Guide.* Circadian Information Limited Partnership, 2010

Posen, David. *The Little Book of Stress Relief.* Firefly books Ltd. New York, NY, 2012

Schwartz, Richard C. *Introduction to the Internal Family Systems Model.* Trailheads Publications, Oak Park, Illinois, 2001

Rothchild, Babette. *8 Keys to Safe Trauma Recovery: Take Charge Strategies to Empower Your Healing*. W.W. Norton. New York and London, 2010

Seppala, Emma, PhD *The Happiness Track*. Harper One, 2016

Siegel, J. Daniel, *Mindsight: The New Science of Personal Transformation*. Bantam Books, New York, NY, 2011

Siegel, D. Ronald. *The Mindfulness Solution, Everyday Practices for Everyday Problems*. The Guildford Press. New York, NY, 2010

Tatkin, Stan. *We Do: Saying Yes to a Relationship of Depth, True Connection, and Enduring Love*. Sounds True. Colorado, 2018

Van Der Kolk, Bessel. *The Body Keeps the Score: Brain, Mind, and Body in the Healing of Trauma*. Viking Penguin, New York, NY, 2014

# ACKNOWLEDGEMENTS

Permissions gratefully acknowledged for all resources shared in this book.

I want to thank my late parents for the privilege of being raised in England, in the western hemisphere, which could have easily been the East, as my father was from East India. That opportunity gave me advantages that I'm grateful to have had, although I may not have recognized and appreciated the value at the time.

Thank you to my Director of Nursing, Judy Watson, for seeing in me something that I did not yet see in myself– an ability to speak about caring for ourselves and others.

Judy supported me in my position as a head nurse in Long Term Care (LTC). This was probably the most challenging and exciting growth opportunity of my nursing career.

For my nursing friends and colleagues from England, Poland and Canada: I have learned so much from you, and

I stand in awe at the depth of caring, laughter and support I have observed and received.

To my teacher, Gary Craig, founder of Emotional Freedom Techniques: I have never met you, but you guided me through countless hours of recordings that helped me get out of my own way to let this gift of healing come through me.

To Dr. Carol Look, a Master EFT trainer: I enjoyed your workshops on trauma, and I thank you for helping to heal parts of my past to increase my capacity to sit with others, and do the work I do.

To Nancy Forrester, MBA, BEd, BSc, Accredited EFT master trainer of trainers in Canada: I am thankful for her friendship as well as mentorship to become an Advanced EFT practitioner.

To Craig Weiner: Thanks for the excellent "Tapping out of Trauma" series.

To Deborah King, a shaman with flair: I appreciate her teaching me how to meditate and how to use my energy as a tool for healing. It's not hard to study in the serene surroundings of Miraval Spa, Tucson, Arizona.

To all of my teachers at Transformational Arts College: I am appreciative and grateful for their insights and wisdom in teaching the acceptance of ourselves as human beings not human "doings." They have helped me to experiment through mindful meditations and body awareness to reach new levels of consciousness of what it means to be on our path in this lifetime and then to serve others to help them discover theirs. Special thanks to Michelle DesRoches, Sue Diplock, Anne-Marie Boudreau, Linda Kuschnir, Joanne Morgan, John Pollard and Ken Sullivan.

To Donna Eden, author of *Energy Medicine for Women* and the *Energies of Love* with her husband, David Feinstein, PhD: My husband and I had the great fortune to join them on an Alaskan cruise and to learn Donna's five-minute energy routine which I still use today to keep my energy protected, in tune and flowing in the right direction.

I thank Dr. Ellyn Bader, PhD, for her amazing year-long on-line program from The Couples Institute.

To Dr. Diane Poole-Heller: I thank her for her teachings on attachment and somatic experiencing program in Boulder Colorado and where I completed the certification program called DARe – The Dynamic Attachment Re-Patterning Experience. Also, for the opportunity to be part of her mastermind therapy group for ongoing support and learning.

Thanks, too, to Ruth Buczynski, PhD, licensed psychologist, President of the National Institute for the Clinical Application of Behavioural Medicine: I am grateful for the updates and the teacher interviews and for the information she shares on the new brain science and fields of therapy.

To my peer group (since graduation): I appreciate your support, especially Sarla, Maria, Lorena and Laura.

I appreciate my hospital work team for all their support, with special thanks to a former manager, Suzanne Henseleit, and former clinical leader, Julie Fischer, for believing in me, offering support and promoting my practice at work.

To Natalie Zlodre, MSW, my supervisor in group trauma work, for her extensive knowledge and her ongoing teaching and support.

And a shout out to my friends, Maureen and Julie, who feed me well and nourish my soul as do their partners, Chris and Gabor.

I thank author Dr. Angela E. Lauria, for supporting my idea to write this book in her intensive writing program at the Author Incubator, Washington, D.C.

And lastly, to my family, without whose support I would never would have got this project off the ground. I thank my husband, Gord, for his patience, ongoing support, and encouragement—it keeps me going. Through his stability and love, he has made me feel safe enough to push through my own boundaries and limiting beliefs to explore and create more of me. And I am forever grateful for that. With love to my eldest daughter, Alisha, and partner John; daughter Rhona and son-in-law David; and the twins, Jannina and Katrina and son-in-law Mark. Also, to my grandchildren, Lexi, Lily and Ruby, who make me laugh and bring such happiness into all of our lives. I feel truly blessed to have you all in my life to experience the joy in learning to open up my heart to love and living this life I get to share with you all.

# ABOUT THE AUTHOR

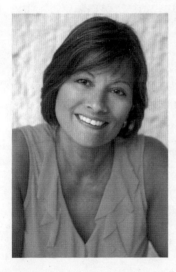

Vij Richards has spent over thirty years in health care, working in ICU/CCU, long term care, and occupational health. Born in England where she did her RN training, she also worked as a nurse in Poland on a construction site before emigrating to Canada. She has worked on the front lines, in management, in the community and in industry. If there is one thing that gives her hope for the future of health care, it is compassion. Compassion for one's self and compassion for others is crucial for us to grow as professionals who are trying to navigate the demands of an ever-changing workplace.

Vij became aware of the stressors at work when, in 2007, the healthy workplace survey at the community hospital where she was employed reported that sixty-eight percent of staff felt stressed on any given day. She felt a need to do something about that—to find a solution.

With awareness and understanding that came from her own experiences, she searched to find a way to make a difference. She went back to school to become a psychotherapist, graduating from Transformational Arts College, Toronto, in 2012.

She now works in a large community hospital, offering emotional support to the staff, and she also has private practices in Milton, Georgetown and Guelph, Ontario, that offer adults counselling for stress, anxiety, depression, loss and trauma. She enjoys living in the country with her husband, Gord, and spending time with her family. When she is not learning, she is travelling and living the life she has created.

Contact Information:
www.miltontherapist.ca

# THANK-YOU

To thank-you for purchasing this book, I am offering you a free ABC handout that gives you the signs for early identification of Compassion Fatigue, suggested ways to balance and choosing to make a commitment to add to your self-care tool box.

You can find the handout on my website: <u>www.milton-therapist.ca</u>.

I wish you all the best in finding ways to cope with the demands of your every day and if this information has touched you in any way, I would love to hear from you.

Your thoughts and ideas are welcome on how to bring nurses together and to better help de-stress so that we can support ourselves strongly, confidently and with compassion.

You can send your stories to: ShiftStress@gmail.com